A Doctor's Prescription for Health Care Reform

The National Medical Association tackles disparities, stigma, and the status quo

Rahn Kennedy Bailey, MD, DFAPA

113th President, National Medical Association

WESTBOW
PRESS
A DIVISION OF THOMAS NELSON

WestBow Press books may be ordered through booksellers or by contacting:

WestBow Press
A Division of Thomas Nelson
1663 Liberty Drive
Bloomington, IN 47403
www.westbowpress.com
1-(866) 928-1240

Cover Photo: Dr. Bailey speaks to a family about their child during a humanitarian trip to Port-Au-Prince, Haiti after the 2010 earthquake. Photo by Janet Caldwell, Meharry Medical College.

ISBN: 978-1-4497-8749-3 (sc)
ISBN: 978-1-4497-8782-0 (e)

Library of Congress Control Number: 2013904361

Printed in the United States of America

WestBow Press rev. date: 6/4/2013

Acknowledgements

This book is a culmination of my 23 years in the medical profession. I greatly appreciate the dedication and tireless hard work of the many people who have supported me throughout the years. This book could not have been produced without the support of my family and colleagues.

First I would like to thank my parents, Sandra Faye Bailey and late Edward Mitchell Bailey. I was raised in a loving and caring home that has made all of my lifelong success possible.

I would like to thank my wife, Theresa Annette Bailey. Her unwavering support and encouragement have been essential to my accomplishments.

To my three children – Candace Alyse, Ebone Brianne and Rahn Mitchell – you have made my world a better place. Your daddy loves you dearly.

Special Thank You

Special thanks should go to my Meharry Medical College leadership team, Wayne J. Riley, MD, President and CEO; and Charles P. Mouton, MD, MS, Senior Vice President for Health Affairs and Dean of the School of Medicine. I appreciate them and everyone in the Meharry family for supporting my work during my NMA presidential year.

Contributions

This book was created with the cooperation and collaboration of the hard working medical professionals at Meharry Medical College, the National Medical Association and others. I would like to thank the following people for their assistance and diligence.

Farzana Alam, MD

Jeffrey A. Barrett, MD

Lalitha Gazula, MD

Osamudiamen Osa-Edoh, MD

Milankumar Nathani, MD

Zohaib Sohail, MD

Dilara Sultana, MD

Michele C. Randle

Darryl R. Matthews, Sr., National Medical Association

Carla Welborn, National Medical Association

Table of Contents

Prologue

Through my years as a physician, friends and colleagues have told me many of stories that drive home the theme of this book – disparities, stigma and access to health care. Some are cautionary tales, but then there are some that are truly sad. Last year, a good friend told me the story of his oldest brother. He was a cross country truck driver, but his company offered no health insurance. My friend's family grew up poor and the thought of health care insurance was an unaffordable luxury. His family depended on over-the-counter medications and when all else failed, the nearest hospital emergency room for health care services.

Whenever my friend's brother became ill, his routine response to seeing a physician was "you know I can't afford that." His brother was supporting a wife and three grandchildren. Insurance simply did not fit in the budget of those daily concerns. While on a cross country drive with pressing deadline to get a load to its destination, my friend's brother started to have chest pains. He had similar chest pains before and they always subsided. Somehow, he felt that these pains were different. Yet, when his wife urged him to go to the hospital during a telephone call, she got the same response – "you know I can't afford that."

Paramedics found him unresponsive in the cab of his truck later that evening. A coroner pronounced him dead at the scene. An autopsy revealed that he died of heart disease, exacerbated by smoking. For my friend's family, the death was sudden and surprising. No one knew about the progression of his disease, even though it was possibly treatable with regular care.

Officially, my friend's brother died of heart disease. In my opinion, he died prematurely because of lack of health insurance. Health care insurance would not have prevented the disease, but it would have provided him the means to routinely seek treatment. A physician would have likely spotted problems on routine examinations. That physician would have provided care to slow the progression of the disease. He could have received treatment without feeling his illness was a financial burden on his family. Multiply what happened to my friend's brother with African-American families across the country who grew up without the means to secure health insurance and access to a doctor. It becomes clear why we have such a wide range of racial health disparities.

The status quo continues to perpetuate these disparities and stigma. Far too many people of all races face the chances of dying without proper medical care. This book is dedicated to changing the fate of people in similar situations as my friend's brother, all of our family members and all Americans. Health care is a right of every American, not only the wealthy or those fortunate enough to have a job that provides health insurance. We hope this book sharpens the debate. After hearing far too many of these stories in my career, in my opinion, it's a debate worthy of our discussion.

CHAPTER 1
Health Care Change That Affects Everyone

Coauthor: B.K. Edmond, MD

In 1895, African-American doctors from across the nation organized to start the National Medical Association (NMA). While members of the NMA have garnered great success and honor as well as access to hospitals across the country, problems African-Americans face in health care persist.

After nearly 120 years, issues of health care disparities and stigma between ethnicities continue. The need for cultural competency is as important now as ever. The arrival of the Patient Protection and Affordable Care Act has the potential of tackling some of the issues that members of the NMA have been concerned about for generations.

The Affordable Care Act is one step – a start – in improving the nation's health care system and making it work for everyone. The National Medical Association will continue to add its voice to the mix of those in the health care field who want to see the system in the United States improve and provide quality care for all of its citizens.

Today, the NMA represents the 37,000 practicing African-American physicians. Gone are the segregated policies that once kept black physicians out of prestigious organizations like the American Medical Association. Gone are the racially exclusive "Jim Crow" laws that dominated employment, housing, transportation, recreation, education and medicine.

The National Medical Association's founding was "conceived in no spirit of racial exclusiveness, fostering no ethnic antagonisms, but born out of the exigency of the American environment…" while extending equal rights and privileges to all physicians.

From the association's beginning, the NMA has led the fight for better medical care and opportunities for all Americans. Its primary focus target health issues related to minority populations and the medically underserved, improving the health status and outcomes of African-Americans and the disadvantaged. From the very beginning, advocacy has been an important part of the NMA. African-American doctors, like blacks in virtually every role in American society who had to fight for basic rights, have always carried the torch of providing quality care, while speaking up against injustices in the system. It is a responsibility members of the NMA take on with pride and determination. It was often the membership's own family members, neighbors and friends they were fighting for, which made that advocacy role very personal. While we continue to advocate for them today, the NMA members understand that their efforts are for all patients, doctors and workers in the health care field. The health care profession, though, is left to deal with the vestiges of the disparities that past discrimination has caused.

African-American doctors represent about three percent of the medical workforce in the country (30,000 out of roughly one million). These physicians, though, are the eyes and ears of many of the poor and indigent patients seeking to access the medical system. The health care system has not worked well for many of these patients. One can argue that the health care system has actually worked against them. As they struggle to receive quality health care, their struggle adversely affects everyone in the health care system. Thus, if the government and health care professionals can improve the system for these patients, it would be a win for everyone who has to access the system at some point.

This book will address three aspects of the health care system – reform, disparities and stigma. These are vitally important issues for the National Medical Association. The NMA has supported the Patient Protection and Affordable Care Act from its inception, in part for these reasons.

It was Dr. Martin Luther King Jr. who said in a 1966 speech to the Medical Committee for Human Rights that of all forms of inequality, "injustice in health care was the most shocking and inhumane." The NMA believes there should not be injustices and disparities in health care. As health care professionals, physicians, nurses and others in the field must make it our professional challenge to end inequities in care because ultimately they create excessive and unwarranted morbidity, and premature and unnecessary death.

The system has not worked well for African-Americans and other minorities. It has become too costly and inequitable. Such has created unfairness. It is the mission of the NMA to advance the art and science of medicine for people of African-American descent, as well as all who are in need through education, advocacy, and the formulation of effective and utility-based health policy.

Talking Disparities

What do we mean when we talk about disparities? Here are a few examples. Prostate cancer results from the development of malignant cells from prostatic tissue, which can result in secondary medical complications and a myriad of psychosocial issues. African-American men bear a disproportionate burden of prostate cancer with regard to incidence and mortality (1).

According to the National Cancer Institute, the incidence and mortality of this disease is higher in African-Americans males in comparison with men from other racial and ethnic groups. Some 60 percent of blacks are more likely to develop prostate cancer and are twice as likely to die from it. Furthermore, some research suggests that the development of prostate cancer in African-American men appears to be more rapid with the probability that more aggressive disease is manifested at an earlier age in this population (1).

Recognizing these devastating statistics, the United States Senate passed a resolution in the summer of 2012 categorizing prostate cancer in African-Americans to have risen to the level of epidemic proportions. Similarly, President Barack Obama proclaimed the month of September as "National Prostate Cancer Awareness Month."

Research has demonstrated that factors such as socioeconomic status, lack of health insurance coverage and inequity of access to health care, are associated with the disproportionate prostate cancer burden on African-American males (1).

With regard to screening methods, there is ongoing controversy about the benefits versus risk/harm from results of Prostate-Specific Antigen (PSA) testing. According to the U.S. Preventive Services Task Force, the medical evidence does not support that the benefits of PSA testing in asymptomatic men outweigh the anticipated side effects resulting in decisions for early treatment which do not lead to a positive outcome. Interventions such as surgery and irradiation can lead to erectile dysfunction, incontinence and even death. The National Cancer Institute is even uncertain that there is enough evidence to determine whether screening by doing a digital rectal exam or performing PSA testing decreases mortality.

However, the debate continues. For the general population, it is recommended that prostate cancer screening begins at age 50 but it is recommended that for African-American males with a first-degree relative with the disease they should discuss annual screening with their doctors at age 40.

One can find similar issues with lung cancer. In 2008, 25.5 percent of non-Hispanic black men smoked compared to 23.6 percent of non-Hispanic white men (2). On average, white men tend to consume more cigarettes (about 30 to 40 percent more) than African-American men. Despite their lower exposure, however, African-American men are 34 percent more likely than white men to develop lung cancer (2).

Black women tend to smoke less than white women do, but the two groups have similar lung cancer rates. Among African-Americans, as with other U.S. population groups, the prevalence of smoking declines as education level increases. Parents can set a positive example for their children by not smoking themselves, and keeping their homes smoke-free (2).

Schools can provide tobacco prevention programs to educate students about the dangers of smoking. States can pass legislation to increase taxes on tobacco products, pass and implement comprehensive smoke-free indoor air quality laws, and limit minors' access to tobacco products.

Another prominent issue today is obesity. Obesity has the potential to cause lifelong problems for a person's general health. For example, more than 80 percent of people with type 2 diabetes are obese (3). Additionally, people who are obese are more likely to develop health issues due to high blood pressure, high cholesterol and physical inactivity. These health issues may contribute to serious illnesses and conditions such as heart disease and stroke (3).

Statistics of obesity rates in African-Americans are greatly alarming. According to Trust for America's Health Report in July 2011, "Facts in Fat: How Obesity Threatens America's Future," over 30 percent of African-American residents living in more than 41 states are obese or overweight. This is in comparison to the fact that there are only four states in which 30 percent or more whites are obese. The Office of Minority Health has found that about four in five African-American women are overweight or obese.

However, adults are not the only ones affected by this epidemic. Data from the Centers for Disease Control and Prevention (CDC) from 2007 through 2010 found that 23.3 percent of African-American boys, aged 6–11, and 24.5 percent African-American girls, ages 6–11 were obese. Clearly, obesity is currently a significant problem within the African-American community that will continue to affect the overall health status of African-Americans for years to come.

Yet another issue is dementia. Dementia is a syndrome of acquired impairment of memory and other cognitive functions caused by structural neuronal damage, which represents a decline of previous level of functioning DSM-IV-TR.

African-Americans are about two times more likely and Hispanics are about one and one-half times more likely than their white counterparts to have Alzheimer's and other dementias (4). Although whites make up the great majority of the more than five million people with Alzheimer's and other dementias, African-Americans and Hispanics are at higher risk for developing the disease.

There are no known genetic factors that can explain the greater prevalence of Alzheimer's and other dementias in African-Americans and Hispanics than in whites. Conditions, such as high blood pressure and diabetes, which are known risk factors for dementias, are more common in African-Americans and Hispanics than in whites (4).

Socioeconomic factors, such as having a low level of education and low income are also associated with greater risk for Alzheimer's and other dementias in all groups. According to Alzheimer News, there are 5.3 million Americans living with the disease and every 70 seconds someone in America develops Alzheimer's disease. By midcentury someone will develop Alzheimer's every 33 seconds. In 2010, there was a half million new cases of Alzheimer's, and in 2050, there will be nearly a million new cases.

Considering Reform

Many African-American physicians continue to choose careers in primary care serving diverse indigenous populations. To this end, the National Medical Association has worked hard to provide a network of support from private and public sources to assist the underserved in accessing quality health care. Regardless of the profession, one will be able to work more efficiently, effectively and with greater skill if health issues are addressed quickly and with little delay as possible. That is the primary advantage of quality health care for individuals.

Currently one in six Americans, roughly 50 million, does not have health insurance (5). As an example, consider the life of a typical single woman, let's call her Jessica, with a child. It has been my experience in working more than 20 years in the health care field that if such an individual walked into my office, there would be at least a one in five chance that she didn't have health insurance – but may still work. This is because four out of five persons without health insurance are employed. Many patients rely on the emergency room for services rather than being seen by a physician on a regular basis. Hypertension, diabetes and other obesity-related diseases can be blunted or treated with lifestyle modifications, screening and overall quality health care. Many do not have access to early care and often find themselves waiting for a disease to progress before seeking help. For example, having your blood pressure checked twice a year can help identify risk of congestive heart failure, heart attacks and strokes.

Jessica, our hypothetical single woman with child, could be anyone in your family. Where did these numbers come from? They emanate from the current health care metric over time. The health care system in the United States was not necessarily planned, but has evolved since its founding. It developed over time into a model in which individuals received quality health care because they had health insurance. Most people had their health insurance because they had gainful employment that provided insurance as an employee benefit. This evolution created a circumstance that left many indigent patients disenfranchised from access to basic health care. For decades, there have been private health care policies and plans provided by insurance companies. Unfortunately, those policies were out of reach financially for many of the working poor and indigent. Basically, if one is unemployed, or only works intermittently, there's a good chance that they will not be able to afford health insurance.

That has resulted in situations whereby many persons who have retired, who are disabled, or who have small children or extended families to support and do not have adequate health insurance. That includes a large percentage of our population, particularly in the economic recession of 2008 when the U.S. work force saw this great contraction and national unemployment nearly reached 10 percent. This was the time that most Americans were living without the safety net of health insurance.

As a physician attempting to treat a patient, it is tragic to recognize that if you had an opportunity to treat him or her earlier you could have done so much more. While working as an intern in internal medicine at a county hospital in Houston, I twice delivered babies in a car parking lot outside the hospital. These women had not received any prenatal care. Neither had her blood pressure checked during pregnancy. Neither had an ultrasound during that time to detect complications in the pregnancy. Missing prenatal care can lead to unwarranted birth defects. Such preventable illnesses can be better addressed with implementation of the Affordable Care Act.

What is the Affordable Care Act (ACA)? It provides greater access to health care for many of the poor and under employed with the help of the federal government. NMA members often take care of people who struggle to take care of themselves. A significant percentage of our NMA members practice medicine in small, solo, or individual medical settings. Thus, the tax breaks for small businesses will help them. Again, these are physicians who frequently take care of patients who are uninsured.

The vehicle to provide the ACA is Medicaid expansion. Individuals or families will be able to earn more annual income, yet still qualify for the Medicaid program. The federal government offers Medicare to all citizens over age 65. It also provides support for about 90 percent of Medicaid funding. Medicaid provides a baseline level of care for the indigent, elderly in nursing homes, and certain children's services.

What are the potential benefits? Let's again consider Jessica and her child after the act has passed. Now there is a very different dynamic. She does not have to be afraid because of lack of health insurance. She now has the flexibility to move to a different location or job. Because of portability, her health insurance will follow her. She will likely go for many of those preventive screenings because they are now free.

In addition, what about Jessica's child? If he had a pre-existing condition like sickle-cell anemia, which is high in the African-American community, he could have been denied health care insurance before the Affordable Care Act. Now, he would be accepted and would be able to receive care under this insurance plan. With the ACA in effect, the system will not preclude this woman and her son from obtaining care because of preexisting conditions. I will explain this in more detail in later chapters. This makes sure more people are in the system, which should help drive down the overall costs of health care.

NMA members also believe the Affordable Care Act dismantles what we consider a two-tier system of health care by equalizing Medicare and Medicaid payments. Some doctors would take Medicaid patients certain days of the week and Medicare and better-paying private-insurance patients other days of the week, limiting time to see the poor. It was a two-tier system, bias based, discrimination laden, which created health care disparities.

Voices against ACA

There are arguments against the Affordable Care Act and those have been voiced loudly in political circles and other doctors. The biggest argument is against the individual mandate, which required all individuals to be covered by health insurances, either by their job or by purchasing their own health insurance. NMA members believe that if everyone pays into the system, then everyone will likely receive better quality care. Everyone may not receive high-level care, but everyone needs to get basic, comprehensive affordable care and preventive services. This will help in many aspects, like driving down high infant mortality rates. Also, if everyone is paying into the system, those who have not seen a doctor before will more than likely be compelled to access the health care system because they are invested in it. Access to the health care system will allow doctors to address preventive and early care with these patients to help prevent future illnesses.

In the end, individuals will still need to take advantage of the new rules created in the Affordable Care Act because there is no better advocate for our health care than ourselves. NMA members believe the Affordable Care Act will allow individuals to do just that without the cloud of financial concerns and fears hanging over their heads. You cannot function in a competitive society if your health care is not in order.

This type of advocacy is nothing for the National Medical Association. The NMA fought against discrimination in health care following World War II, helping force hospitals and medical schools to gradually admit African-American students. The number of black students enrolled in medical schools increased 31 percent in 1955-56. The NMA lobbied to pass the Civil Rights Act of 1964 and supported Dr. Martin Luther King's 1965 voter-registration campaign in Selma, Ala., which outlawed discrimination in government-funded health programs. The NMA was the first medical group in 1965 to support Medicare. President Lyndon B. Johnson spoke to the NMA in 1968 to thank the association and tout the success of Medicare.

President Johnson said in his address to the NMA on Aug. 14, 1968 that many predicted the ruin of medicine in America because of Medicare.

"I remember one particular critic who said that on the first day of Medicare, 'A line of patients will stretch all the way from Chicago to Kansas City,' " President Johnson said. "But these prophets of doom about Medicare were just as wrong as they were about social security... Medicare is working its wonders. It is saving lives. It is replacing fear and anguish with confidence and with serenity. And our older citizens are now getting medical care, not as charity cases any more, not on hand-outs from their sons-in-law, but as insured, equal patients. In short, Medicare is an expression of fundamental humanity. In short, Medicare is a triumph of rightness."

Look at how many people are supportive of Medicare today and how many would argue taking it away. I believe the same would take place once the Affordable Care Act has taken hold.

Through the upcoming chapters, I use numerous issues I have faced as a psychiatrist to address the issues of reform, disparities and stigma. While much of the content within these chapters is derived from my medical writing, selected ones are highlighted to emphasize our key themes in hopes to address the NMA efforts to improve the U.S. health care system for all.

References

1. Fact Sheet. Cancer Health Disparities. National Cancer Institute website. http://www.cancer.gov/cancertopics/factsheet/disparities/cancer-health-disparities

2. Facts and Figures. Smoking Rates Among African-Americans. American Lung Association website. http://www.lung.org/stop-smoking/about-smoking/facts-figures/african-americans-and-tobacco.html

3. Obesity-Related Diseases. Understanding Obesity. ObesityinAmerica.org. Chevy Chase, Md. http://www.obesityinamerica.org/understandingObesity/diseases.cfm

4. New Report Says African-Americans and Hispanics More Likely to have Alzheimer's disease than Whites. Alzheimer News, March 9, 2010. http://www.alz.org/news_and_events_18984.asp

5. Christie L., Number of People Without Health Insurance Climb. CNN Money. Sept. 13, 2011. http://money.cnn.com/2011/09/13/news/economy/census_bureau_health_insurance/index.htm

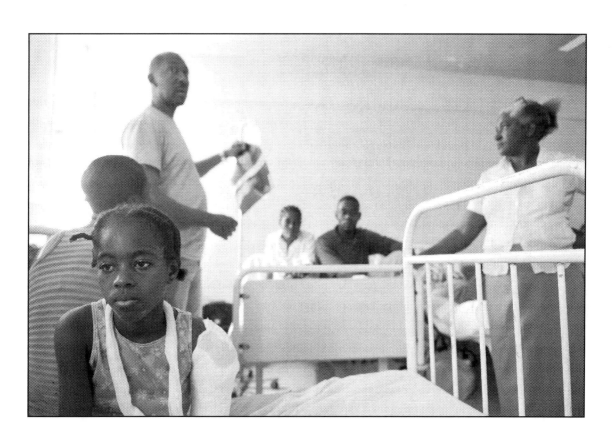

Dr. Bailey addresses patients and health care workers at a hospital in Haiti in late January, 2010 after the Haitian earthquake. Photo by Janet Caldwell, Meharry Medical College.

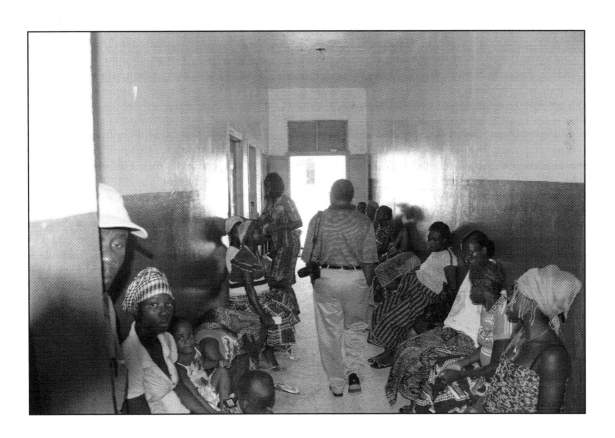

Liberian patients crowd a narrow hallway in John F. Kennedy Hospital in Monrovia, Liberia in hopes to see a physician. Liberia ranks next to last among countries with the fewest doctors per population.

CHAPTER 2

Why the Affordable Care Act Matters

Coauthor: William D. Richie, MD, FAPA

On June 28, 2012, the United States Supreme Court upheld the constitutionality of the "Patient Protection and Affordable Care Act (PPACA)" – a health care reform law. Health care reform is a general term used for discussing major health policy creation or changes. This health care reform actually refers to two, separate pieces of legislation:

The Patient Protection and Affordable Care Act was adopted on March 23, 2010. The goal of the initiative was to make the health care system more efficient and more accessible. In this article authors discussed on issues with current health system and highlights of Affordable Care Act.

Issues with the Current U.S. Health System

In 2006, the U.S. census reported that 46 million Americans (recently revised downward to 45 million) have no health insurance. In addition, more than nine million children lack health insurance in America. Some 18,000 people die each year because they are uninsured (1).

Disparities in Access to Health Care

In the current health system there are several disparities which need attention. Ethnic minorities receive less preventive care. As compare to others, this minority population has less access to specialists. This population has also been offered fewer expensive and technical procedures than non-ethnic minorities (2).

Reasons for Disparities to Health Care Access

In order to improve U.S. health care system, it is critical to know the reasons for disparities in health care access. These reasons include lack of insurance coverage, lack of regular source of care and lack of financial resources. In addition, structural barriers such as poor transportation, health literacy, age, stigma and lack of cultural competence by health care provider are also important to note.

Fairness

Over one-third (36 percent) of families living below the poverty line are uninsured. Hispanic Americans (34 percent) are more than twice as likely to be uninsured as white Americans, (13 percent), while 21 percent of black Americans have no health insurance (3).

Sustainability

Half of all bankruptcies are caused by medical bills. Three-quarters of those filings are people with health insurance. U.S. health care spending is approximately $2 trillion per year or $6,697 per person (More than any other developed country in the world) (4).

Quality

United States leads the world in spending on health care, "countries spending substantially less than the US have healthier populations. For example, the infant mortality rate for the U.S. is now higher than for many other industrial countries (5).

Consequences of Being Uninsured

The uninsured would most likely miss the preventive and routine care for chronic conditions. If these chronic conditions are not treated on time, it is likely that the uninsured patient would incur extended financial risks. In addition, these patients would end up hospitalized frequently for conditions that are potentially avoidable. Ultimately the communities will pay a price for the gaps in health insurance coverage of their residents (6).

Affordable Care Act Highlights

The Affordable Care Act was signed into law on March 23, 2010. Future goals for this Act is to provide access to over 30 million uninsured people, make health care more affordable by giving tax credits to those that needs it and reduce the cost to individuals and government by encouraging integrated care. Key Provisions in the Affordable Care Act include the following: are increasing Medicaid eligibility to 133 percent of the federal poverty line population, requiring large employers (have up to 50 employees) to provide affordable insurance to employees, creating an insurance market (exchange) and overall health insurance reform (7).

ACA Benefits

ACA benefits patients through provisions that will help more children get health care coverage and allow younger adults the opportunity to stay on their parent's health care insurance until age 26. The ACA also gives patients access to recommended preventative services without cost. The law prevents insurance companies from placing annual limits on health care and end lifetime caps. Through the ACA, insurance companies must cover preexisting conditions and provide medications at cheaper prices (8).

Physicians will also benefit from ACA through Medicare payment changes, a 10 percent incentive payment for primary care physicians, a 10 percent incentive payment for general surgeons performing major surgery in health professional shortage areas, a five percent incentive payment for mental health services and increased geographic payment adjustments. ACA should also extend the incentive payment for Medicare quality reporting (9). Overall benefits of ACA are described in Table 1.

Table 1

• Promoting the ACA initiative will allow more young people to stay on their parents' health plans.
• Millions of uninsured Americans will receive health care coverage.
• No one can be denied coverage because of pre-existing conditions.

• Insurance companies will also be unable to drop people just because they get sick.
• Insurance companies would also be obliged to pay a greater percentage of a patient's premium for medical care than they would in the past.
• There would be more money in the ACA for prevention than existed in the past.
• There would be more money for care coordination than existed in the past.
• There would be greater commitment to innovation than ever before.
• There would be a greater commitment, with incentives - to pay for and reward quality, rather than volume - than existed in the past.
• The states continue to prepare for setting up insurance exchanges; even the states that have filed suit against the ACA are working to implement it.
• dual eligible (those eligible for Medicare and Medicaid) now have a whole office focused on coordinating their care; improving their health outcomes, and saving the system money

Why Defend the ACA, June 2012

Supreme Court Ruling on Affordable Care Act

In March 2012, the U.S. Supreme Court considered the following questions regarding the constitutionality of ACA. Two critical questions centered around the individual mandate, that portion of the law which requires individuals to purchase health insurance. If an individual does not comply, they must pay the tax.

- Is the individual mandate unconstitutional?
- If the individual mandate is unconstitutional, should the rest of ACA fall with it?

The Supreme Court was also asked if states could be forced to expand their Medicaid rolls. And if a tax could be levied for not having insurance before it takes effect?

On June 28, 2012, the Supreme Court upheld the constitutionality of ACA. The individual mandate was upheld. The Supreme Court also held that the Anti-Injunction Act (prohibits challenging a tax before it is paid) does not apply and the court could decide the merits. Furthermore, Medicaid expansion was limited but upheld and Congress cannot revoke a state's entire medical funding if that state refuses to participate in Medicaid expansion. The state's choice of non-compliance would only impact new funds (10).

Other key provisions to be implemented with the individual mandate are: coverage to anyone regardless of health status; people in the same age group pay the same premium regardless of health status; every company with workforce of more than 50 full-time-equivalent employees would offer affordable health insurance to its employees (11).

Conclusion

While there are many debatable points of the Affordable Care Act, overall, the NMA believes health care reform is indeed a major piece of legislation which when fully implemented will greatly change the country's current health care system. While the implementation will require refining, it is a necessary change to establish more efficient U.S. health care system that provides more access to care and reduce the disparities.

References

1. The Impact of Health Insurance Coverage on Health Disparities in the United States, Human Development Report, UNDP, 2005; The Great Divide: When Kids Get Sick, Insurance Matters, Families USA Publication No. 07-102, February 2007; Insuring America's Health: Principles and Recommendations, Institute of Medicine, January 2004)

2. Fiscella, K et al., (2000). Inequality in quality: Addressing socioeconomic, racial, and ethnic disparities in health care. JAMA; 283(19), 2579-2584. Kaiser Commission on Medicaid and the Uninsured (KCMU), "The Uninsured and Their Access to Health Care" (December 2003). G. E. Fryer, S. M. Dovey, and L. A. Green, "The Importance of Having a Usual Source of Health Care," American Family Physician 62 (2000): 477. Agency for Healthcare Research and Quality (AHRQ), "National Healthcare Disparities Report," U.S. Department of Health and Human Services (July 2003)

3. The Impact of Health Insurance Coverage on Health Disparities in the United States, Human Development Report, UNDP, 2005.

4. Illness and Injury as Contributors to Bankruptcy," Himmelstein et al, Health Affairs, February 2, 2005. Catlin, A, et al, "National Health Spending in 2005." Health Affairs 26:1 (2006).

5. The Impact of Health Insurance Coverage on Health Disparities in the United States, Human Development Report, UNDP, 2005

6. Kirby JB et al, 2010 Nov; 47(4):1035-51. PMID: 21308569. Kozak L.J, 2001. "Trends in Avoidable Hospitalizations, 1980–1998." Health Affairs 20(2):225-232.

7. www.healthcare.gov

8. Paul Fronstin and Bill Erwin, The Alliance for Health Reform Sourcebook Covering Health Issues, 6th Edition (2011 Update) Chapter 4 – Employer-Sponsored Health Coverage, June 13, 2011 www.healthcare.gov

9. www.hsreform.org

10. Highlights of Supreme Court Ruling on Affordable Care Act. SuccessEHS -June 28, 2012

11. Sally P. Schreiber, Alistair M. Nevius. Supreme Court Upholds Health Care Law. Journal of Accountancy: June 28, 2012.

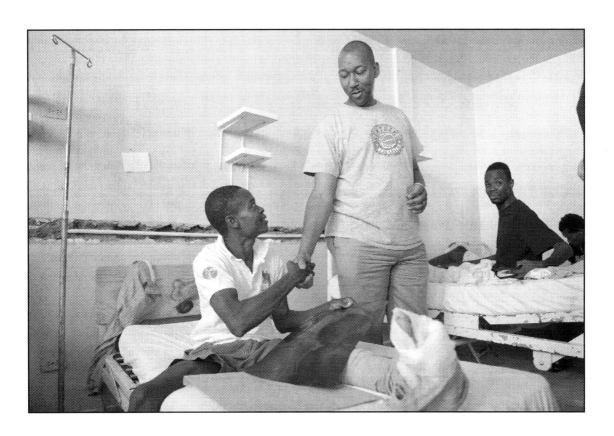

Dr. Bailey shakes hands and comforts a young patient who broke his leg during the 2010 earthquake. Photo by Janet Caldwell, Meharry Medical College.

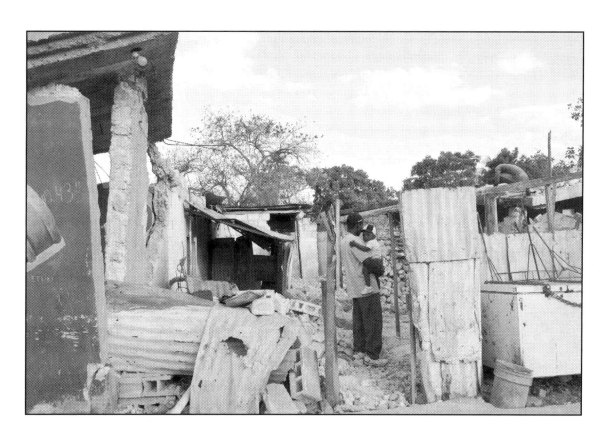

A man holds his son while viewing the devastation around him in Port-Au-Prince, Haiti.
Photo by Janet Caldwell, Meharry Medical College.

CHAPTER 3

The Voice of Black Doctors
on Reform: A Survey

Physicians are key players in health care and understanding their opinions regarding health care is crucial, especially considering the inevitable, impending changes to the U.S. health care system. The creators of a recent questionnaire administered at the 2012 National Medical Association convention sought to discover what physicians, as well as other allied health professionals and stakeholders, thought about health care reform, especially in response to the U.S. Supreme Court's ruling on June 28, 2012 to uphold the constitutionality of the Patient Protection and Affordable Care Act. The Physicians' Beliefs and U.S. Health Care Reform Questionnaire was conducted in person at the National Medical Association's annual convention in New Orleans, La. from Monday, July 30 through Wednesday, Aug. 1, 2012.

Methods and Procedures

The questionnaire was developed with approximately 30 items to be answered on a five-point Likert scale. It was administered at the National Medical Association's annual Convention and & Scientific Assembly in New Orleans, La. from July 30 through Aug. 1, 2012. Each survey respondent was asked to think about the way U.S. health care reform could affect their lives, as well as how they felt about the Supreme Court Ruling on the Patient Protection and Affordable Care Act (ACA). The questionnaire was handed out during session meetings and in central locations such as the sitting areas and exhibition hall of the Ernest N. Morial Convention Center. The center was frequented by NMA convention attendees. Questions were asked based on a Likert Scale with 1 being designated as "Strongly Agree," 2 as "Agree," 3 as "Neither Agree or Disagree," 4 as "Disagree," and 5 as "Strongly Disagree." Either one or two surveyors approached attendees to ask for their cooperation in completing the questionnaire. Each survey took from 10 to 20 minutes to complete.

Research Population

The benefit was to have access to a large number of people in attendance who are members of the National Medical Association, the largest and oldest national organization representing African-American physicians and their patients. The convention was open to any medical professional including physicians, scientists, nurse practitioners, physician assistants, nurses, dieticians, administrators, students and other professionals working in health care. Each survey respondent was asked to think about the way U.S. health care reform could affect their lives, as well as how they felt about the U.S. Supreme Court ruling on the Patient Protection and Affordable Care Act (ACA). The survey was designed to collect the following information from our target population: gender, country of origin, area of practice, years in practice, type of practice and location of practice (city, suburb, or rural).

Results

As of Tuesday July 31, 2012, there were more than 3,000 people officially registered for the National Medical Association Convention and 270 attendees completed the survey. The survey has a 4.8 percent error level at the 90 percent confidence interval, a 5.7 percent error level at the 95 percent confidence interval, and a 7.5 percent error level at the 99 percent confidence interval.

Demographics
Gender

Among the 270 attendees who completed the survey, 44 percent (n = 120) were female and 52 percent (n = 140) were male. 4 percent (n=10) of the respondents failed to answer. (See Figure 1)

Figure 1. *Survey Demographics: Gender*

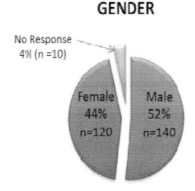

Countries of Origin

The respondents were very diverse and came from a variety of backgrounds. Respondents came from many different countries of origin, such as the United States, Jamaica, Ghana and the Bahamas. (See Table 1)

Table 1. Survey Demographics: Country of Origin

USA	British West Indies
Jamaica	Pakistan
Ghana	Bermuda
Bahamas	Barbados
Trinidad & Tobago	Caribbean
Panama	West Indies
United Kingdom	

Specialties Represented

The respondents also represented many areas of medicine. There were physicians and residents from both primary care and specialties. (See Table 2) There were also respondents who self-identified as medical students, externs, physician assistants, health administrators, and non-physician health care administrators.

Table 2. *Survey Demographics: Specialties Represented*

Emergency Medicine	Family Medicine	Internal Medicine
Internal Medicine/Pediatrics	Pediatrics	Surgery
Psychiatry	Radiation Oncology	Radiology
Obstetrics/Gynecology	Addiction Medicine	Endocrinology
Rheumatology	Ophthalmology	Urology
Neurology	Gastroenterology	Preventive Medicine
Anesthesiology	Pain Medicine	Oncology
Allergy	Public Health	Occupational Medicine
Otolaryngology	Cardiology	Physical Medicine & Rehabilitation
Dermatology	**OTHER** Resident, Extern, Medical Student	Physician Assistant Health Administrator Non Physician Health Care Provider

Years in Practice

Many of the respondents for the survey had been practicing for more than 30 years. They were followed by physicians who had been practicing for 20–25 years, 15–20 years, and 25–30 years. (See Table 3)

Table 3. *Survey Demographics: Years in Practice*

YEARS IN PRACTICE	# OF RESPONDENTS
Less than 1 years	8
1 – 5 years	16
5 – 10 years	17
10 – 15 years	28
15 – 20 years	38
20 – 25 years	40
25 – 30 years	37
30 + years	53
Retired	6
NA	17
No Response	10

Type of Practice

Most of the respondents for the survey were part of a group practice. Other respondents were part of a solo practice or a hospital practice. This was followed by partnership, academic, other, or no response. (See Figure 2)

Table 4. Survey Demographics: Type of Practice

Type of Practice	# of Respondents
Solo	66
Group	73
Hospital	61
Partnership	18
Academic	2
Other	14
No Response	19
NA	17

Location of Practice

The majority of the respondents were from cities, while only a few were from areas they would call suburban or rural. Some respondents had mixed practices and were in both cities and rural areas, while others were in both city and suburban areas. *(See Figure 3)*

Location of Practice

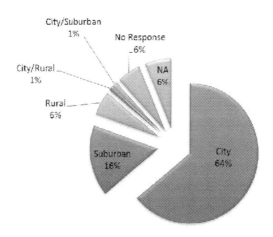

Survey Responses – A Preliminary Review

Strongly Agree

Results from survey show that 95.47 percent of the respondents agreed with the Supreme Court's decision to uphold the Constitutionality of the Affordable Care Act. (Strongly Agree = 203, Agree = 50, Neither Agree Nor Disagree = 6, Disagree = 5, Strongly Disagree = 1. 5 did not respond)

The survey also found that 88.59 percent of the respondents agreed that the ACA would increase access to care. (Strongly Agree = 110, Agree = 123, Neither Agree Nor Disagree = 14, Disagree = 12, Strongly Disagree = 4. 7 respondents did not respond.)

Some 96.23 percent of the respondents agreed that they were relieved that all health plans would be required to accept all patients with respect to their pre-existing conditions. In general, most physicians support this provision of the ACA. (Strongly Agree = 174, Agree = 81, Neither Agree Nor Disagree = 8, Disagree = 2, Strongly Disagree = 0, No response = 5)

To the question on whether or not they respondents were hopeful for the future of health care in the U.S. due to the Affordable Care Act, 78.57 percent indicated that they agreed that they were hopeful for the future of health care in the US due to the ACA. (Strongly Agree = 87, Agree = 122, Neither Agree Nor Disagree = 34, Disagree = 17, Strongly Disagree = 6, No response = 4)

Strongly Disagree

There were some points in which the respondents disagreed with the statements. One of these was about their general thoughts about the U.S. health care system in general and 80 percent disagreed that they were considering leaving medicine due to current issues within the health care system of the U.S. (Strongly Agree = 7, Agree = 13, Neither Agree Nor Disagree = 31, Disagree = 79, Strongly Disagree = 133, No response = 7)

Another item respondents disagreed on was regarding the Supreme Court's decision to uphold the constitutionality of the Affordable Care Act. Some 90.5 percent disagreed and were not disappointed with the decision. (Strongly Agree = 3, Agree = 9, Neither Agree Nor Disagree = 13, Disagree = 63, Strongly Disagree = 175, No Response = 7)

Conclusion

Overall, most NMA physicians who answered the survey had favorable opinions regarding the Patient Protection and Affordable Care Act. However, the opinions varied over the more specific provisions and there was no consensus on the deeper issues. Further study of physician opinions regarding the ACA may be necessary. While most respondents agreed that it is a good first step and are hopeful, it is important to note that many physicians worry about the future of health care in the United States. These physicians hope that the progress for inclusiveness of basic, quality care for all patients, regardless of perceived barriers, will continue.

References

1. Lowes, Robert. (6/28/2012). Supreme Court Upholds Affordable Care Act. Medscape Medical News. Retrieved from http://www.medscape.com/viewarticle/765416 on July 2, 2012.
2. Meyer, Harris. (6/28/2012). What the Supreme Court Decision Really Means to Doctors. Medscape Business of Medicine. Retrieved from http://www.medscape.com/viewarticle/766583 on July 2, 2012.
3. Fiore, Marrecca and John E. McDonough, DPh, MPA. (6/28/2012). ACA Future Uncertain? 'Equally Potent Threats Lie Ahead'. Medscape Internal Medicine. Retrieved from http://www.medscape.com/viewarticle/766599?sssdmh=dm1.798516&src=nldne on July 2, 2012.
4. Brauser, Deborah. (6/28/2012). Mental Health Organizations Weigh in On ACA Ruling. Medscape Medical News. Retrieved from http://www.medscape.com/viewarticle/766600?sssdmh=dm1.798 516&src=nldne on July2, 2012.

5. Pho, Kevin. (March 26, 2012). Despite Flaws, Health Care Law is Needed. CNN. Retrieved from http://www.cnn.com/2012/03/25/opinion/pho-health-reform/index.html on July 3, 2012.

6. Health Resources and Services Administration. Affordable Care Act Update. US Department of Health and Human Services. Retrieved from http://www.hrsa.gov/about/affordablecareact/index.html on July 3, 2012.

7. Moffit, Robert. (June 19, 2010.) Obamacare and its Impact on Doctors. Wall Street Journal. Retrieved from http:// online.wsj.com/article/SB100014240527487041229045731521352501839 0.html on July 3, 2012.

8. Kocher, Robert MD and Ezekiel J. Emanuel, MD, Nancy-Ann M. DeParle, JD. (October 19, 2010). The Affordable Care Act and the Future of Clinical Medicine: The Opportunities and Challenges. *Annals of Internal Medicine*. 153(8):536-9. Epub 2010 Aug 23.

9. Goldman, John M. MD. (January 18, 2011). Comments on the Affordable Care Act and the Future of Clinical Medicine. *Annals of Internal Medicine*. Vol. 154(2):140-141.

10. Sommers, Benjamin D. MD, PhD and Andrew B. Bindman, MD. (April 25, 2012) New Physicians, the Affordable Care Act, and the Changing Practice Of Medicine. *Journal of the American Medical Association* .Vol 307(16): 1697-1698.

11. Jacobson, Peter D. JD, MPH and Shelley A. Jazowski, BA. (August 2011) Physicians, The Affordable Care Act, and Primary Care: Disruptive Change or Business as Usual? *Journal of General Internal Medicine. Vol 26(8):934-7. Epub 2011 Apr 1.*

12. Tieman, J. (March-April 2012) Physicans and the Affordable Care Act: Much To Like. *Health Progress*. Vol 93 (3): 61-2.

13. National Medical Association. (2012) About Us – Overview. National Medical Association. Retrieved from http://www.nmanet.org/index.php?option=com_content&view=article&id=1 &Itemid=2 on July 3, 2012.

14. Survey Findings: Physician's Attitudes on the Affordable Care Act. *Jackson Health Care*. Retrieved from http://www.jacksonhealthcare.com/media-room/surveys/physician-attitudes-on-the-affordable-care-act-2012.aspx

15. Collins SR, Robertson R, Garber T, Doty MM. (April 2012). Tracking Trends in Health System Performance: Gaps in Health Insurance: Why So Many Americans Experience Breaks in Coverage And How the Affordable Care Act will help: Findings from the Commonwealth Fund Health Insurance Tracking Survey of US Adults. 2011. *Issue Brief (Commonwealth Fund)*. Vol 9:1 – 22.

16. Mitchell CD, Truitt MS, Shifflette VK, Johnson V, Mangram AJ, Dunn EL. (March 2012). Who Will Cover the Cost of Undocumented Immigrant Trauma Care? *Journal of Trauma and Acute Care Surgery*.Vol 72(3): 609-612.

17. _____. (March 29, 2012) New Survey: 75% of Physicians Largely Oppose the Affordable Care Act, The President's Healthcare Law. *Tom Coburn, MD. United States Senator from Oklahoma*. Retrieved from http://www.coburn.senate.gov/public/index.cfm/ pressreleases?ContentRecord_id=11cb14a2-2482-451e-8805-e59bd33fb55b on July 3, 2012.

18. Antiel, Ryan A. M.A., Farr A. Curlin, M.D., Katherine M. James, M.P.H., and Jon C. Tilburt, M.D., M.P.H. (October 1, 2009) Physician's Beliefs and US Health Care Reform – A National Survey. *The New England Journal of Medicine*.Vol. 361:e23

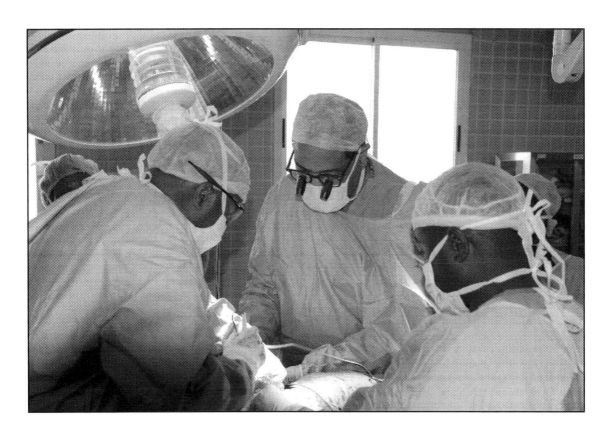

Physicians from the National Medical Association perform an operation at a hospital in Liberia. NMA members perform numerous operations and taught medical classes during a 2013 mission.

CHAPTER 4
A Case for Open Access

Coauthor: Candace Bailey, BS

Numerous research studies have documented differences in access and use of health care services for minority populations compared with the general population. One of the nation's health goals, as described by former U.S. Surgeon General Dr. David Satcher, must be the elimination of racial and ethnic disparities in health status. These discrepancies have been documented repeatedly over the years across a board range of medical conditions.

Such inconsistencies have existed despite improvements in health and availability of newer medications for the nation as a whole. The concern for open access has clinical, ethical and political implications. This chapter will particularly focus on these disproportions, delineating and addressing the issues related to limitations in access to health care. Consequently, this chapter will identify strategies to improve access, promote appropriate use and enhance the quality of health care for all Americans.

The Dilemma

America's medical system has reached a dilemma in addressing the health care needs of ethnic minorities. The reasons behind these disparities are not so well understood. This problem has emerged from a historic and social context in which health care has been differentially allocated on the basis of social class, race and ethnicity. Remnants of this history continue to harmfully affect the current framework of health care delivery. Relevant data suggests that African-Americans have less access to care, receive inferior care frequently and at times are recipients of seemingly bias clinical judgments based primarily on their race. The complexity of the causes of these disparities is difficult to fully appreciate, but they largely reflect socio-economic differences, differences in health-related risk factors, environmental degradation, and direct and indirect consequences of discrimination in the implementation of the American health care system.

Crossing the threshold of skepticism will require a comprehensive approach. First, physicians must become keenly aware that these differences exist. Next, productive change will require an active and concerted effort by those individuals who advocate for quality health care for all patients. That is particularly the care for those who are socioeconomically disenfranchised. Finally, it is becoming increasingly apparent, that an initiative such as this will require the leadership and support of professional medical organizations.

Factors that influence racial and ethnic disparities

There are three factors can play a part in health care disparities – the health care plan, the provider or the patient. Any one of these factors can skew treatments and provide the patient with a less than optimal outcome. The challenge is that there are times that two or even all three of these factors are in play. It is critical for health care professionals to be aware of these cultural differences and bring in a sensitivity to them that will help knock down those barriers that can result in health care disparities.

Health care plans

Characteristics of health care systems and the legal and regulatory context of health care delivery are potential sources of inequalities in treatment. Many of these racial and ethnic differences are due to socioeconomic factors. Rates of health insurance vary greatly among racial and ethnic groups. Minorities are more likely to be enrolled in more affordable, but "low-end" health plans (1). This is due to fewer or lack of resources per patient and stricter limits on covered services. It was reported that racial and ethnic minorities are less likely than whites to possess health insurance (2). They are more likely to be beneficiaries of publicly funded health insurance, e.g. Medicaid (3).

A recent study involving depressed Medicaid recipients found that despite the easy availability of effective treatments, African-Americans were less likely than whites to receive an antidepressant at the time of their initial depression diagnosis. Consequently, of those receiving an antidepressant, whites were more likely than African-Americans to receive selective serotonin reuptake inhibitors (SSRIs) versus tricyclic antidepressants (TCAs)(4). SSRIs are newer, better and better-tolerated antidepressants than TCAs. Another study involving Medicare managed care patients showed that African-Americans are less likely to receive important components of clinical care such as follow-up after hospitalization for mental illness, diabetic eye exams, breast cancer screenings and beta blockers after heart attacks (5).

The Health Care Provider

Three mechanisms might be operative in producing discriminatory pattern of health care from the provider's side of the exchange. Those are:

*Bias (or prejudice) against minorities;

*Greater clinical uncertainty when interacting with minority patients;

*Beliefs (or stereotypes) held by the provider about the behavior or health of minorities (6).

Based on some evidence, physicians may contribute to differences in care by being biased and prejudiced in the physical evaluation of an ill minority patient. In the 1999 article by Schulman and colleagues, they reported vast differences in physicians' decisions to refer patients for cardiac catheterization. This study involved black and white actors playing roles of patients exhibiting and presenting the same symptoms of heart disease. They found that black women were significantly less likely than white men to be recommended for such a referral (7).

Uncertainty about a patient's condition can result, as well as enhance disparities of treatment. If physicians are having difficulty in making a diagnosis since symptoms are not clear cut, they may tend to put an emphasis on prior beliefs about the patient based on age, gender, socioeconomic status, race or ethnicity. This opens the possibility that medical decisions and the course of treatment will reflect the subjective variability and preferences of the physician (8, 9).

Time pressures, resource constraints, complex thinking and decision-making involved in every medical encounter, have been identified as conditions that may increase the likelihood that stereotyping will occur. This is due to the need for cognitive "short cuts" and limit information to adequately assess patients. For instance, as the 1990 General Social Survey (GSS) revealed that whites viewed blacks more negatively relative to whites on a number of dimensions including, propensity towards violence (50 percent rated blacks as more prone to violence) and preference for living on public assistance (78 percent rated blacks as preferring to live off welfare as compared with whites)(10).

The Patient

Patient reactions during a medical encounter may influence and contribute to disparities in health care. Treatment plans recommended by a health care provider may either be accepted or refused by a patient. A small number of studies suggest that racial and ethnic minorities are more likely to refuse treatment (11, 12, 13). Contributory factors can also include trust in the clinician, preferences for treatment type and outcome, information and understanding about the patient's condition and any perception of discrimination in health care settings.

Language and culture are essential in the delivery of health care. Cultural or linguistic barriers crucially affect the quality of health care. In 1990, 14 million Americans were not English-proficient, according to the U.S. Census. In a recent survey, physicians reported that more than half of their patients did not follow medical treatments because of this barrier.

Scopes of open access

Open access is the idea/entity that the best quality of medical care has clinical, ethnic and political implications. It is the duty of every physician to "first do no harm" (primum non nocere). This duty reflects that all physicians will render the best quality of care and treatment to each patient. With the current era of the health care delivery system and rising health care costs, deference to physician autonomy has been restricted if not diminished. Another point is that every patient differs in a wide variety of demographics as to age, gender, sex and race. For instance, African-Americans are more likely to respond better to thiazide diuretics compared to Caucasians or the general population. One study noted that ethnic disparities exist in antipsychotic prescription patterns among a large number of publicly insured patients treated for schizophrenia (14).

Politically, the issue of open access addresses the historical complexity of the basic mistrust that many in the African-American community have maintained over generations, and even centuries, for the American organized health care system. The most striking example of this mistrust is related to the "Tuskegee Study of Untreated Syphilis in the Negro Male" trial that began in 1932 (15, 18).

In 1932, the Public Health Service, working with the Tuskegee Institute, began a study to record the natural history of syphilis in hopes of justifying treatment programs for blacks. It was called the "Tuskegee Study of Untreated Syphilis in the Negro Male" (12). Researchers told men involved in the study that they were being treated for "bad blood," a local term used to describe several ailments, including syphilis, anemia, and fatigue.

In truth, they did not receive the proper treatment needed to cure their illness. Although originally projected to last six months, the study actually went on for 40 years. Once news broke, it brought a chilling effect on African-Americans participating in medical studies (19). While the need for blacks to participate in medical studies is critical today, the "Tuskegee Study" and its aftermath continues to create fear in blacks not only of medical trials, but of the health care system in general.

This history have caused many to question and criticize the U.S. health care system. It not only precludes open access for the most effective treatments and medications, but also undermines the physician-patient relationship. Minorities and the chronically mentally ill are traditionally the most disenfranchised from open access medical care.

This scenario is particularly important now, in that we as a psychiatric profession find ourselves at a most exciting time in our collective research history. We now have new generation medications that offer the prospects of better clinical outcomes, fewer troublesome adverse side effects, as well as the renewed opportunity to more effectively treat certain psychiatric conditions which have hitherto been very difficult to treat. A new study confirmed that use of the newer medications to treat mental illness is cost-effective, despite the drugs' initial high expense (16). The research showed that overall health care costs decreased in the year after starting an atypical antipsychotic, with patients exhibiting significant clinical improvements.

In essence, implementation of effective strategies and interventions to promote the use of "evidence-based" guidelines would be necessary to reduce disparities in health care. These strategies would consist of community-based health care workers, minority health care providers and interpreters (17). Making information available to patients by providing books, pamphlets and in-person instructions will increase patients' knowledge on how to best access care, encourage them to ask the right questions during clinical encounters and intensify their participation in treatment decisions (17). Consequently, a call for future research concentrating on identifying appropriate priorities such as the influence of bias, prejudice, stereotyping and clinical uncertainty of health care providers including inquiries into the importance of cultural competence and health care disparities will certainly improve health care for ethnic and racial minority populations (17).

References

1. National Academy of Sciences, Confronting the Causes of "Unequal Treatment." Accessed from www4.nas.edu, 2002

2. Collins, K.S, Hall A. and Neuhaus, C. U.S. Minority Health: A Chartbook. New York: The Commonwealth Fund.

3. The Henry J. Kaiser Family Foundation. (2000). Key Facts: Kaisser Commission on Medicaid and the Uninsured. Accessed from the Internet site www.kff.ort. June 18, 2001.

4. Melfi, C.A., Croghan, T.W., Hanna, et al: Racial Variation in Antidepressant Treatment in a Medicaid Population. Journal of Clinical Psychiatry 61:1, 16-21, 2000.

5. Schneider, E.C., Zaslavsky, A.M.; and Epstein, A.M.: Racial Disparities in the Quality of Care for Enrollees in Medicare Managed Care. Journal of American Medical Association, 287:10, 1288-1294, 2002.

6. Balsa, A., and McGuire, T.G. "Prejudice, Uncertainty and Stereotypes as Sources of Healthcare Disparities," Boston University, unpublished manuscript, 2001.

7. Schulman, K.A., Berlin, J.A., Harless, W., et all: The effect of race and sex on physicians' recommendation for cardiac catheterization. New England Journal of Medicine, 340: 618-626, 1999.

8. Eisenberg, J.M. Doctors' Decisions and the Costs of Medical Care. Ann Arbor, Michigan. Health Care Administration Press. 1986.

9. Wennberg, J.E., Understanding geographic variations in health care delivery. New England Journal of Medicine. 340(1); 32-39, 1999.

10. 1990 General Social Survey.

11. Canto. J.G., Allison, J.J., Kiefe, C.I., et al: Relations of race and sex to the use of reperfusion therapy in Medicare beneficiaries with acute myocardial infarction. The New England Journal of Medicine, 2000; 342:1094-1100.

12. Sedlis, S.P., Fisher, V.J., Tice, D. et al: Racial differences in performance of invasive cardiac procedures in a Department of Veterans Affairs Medical Center. Journal of Clinical Epidemiology, 1997; 50(8): 899-901.

13. Schecter, A.D., Goldschmidt-Clermong, P.J. McKee, G. et al: Influence of gender, race and education on patient preferences and recipient of cardiac catheterizations among coronary care unit patients. American Journal of Cardiology, 1996; 78(9): 996-1001.

14. Kuno E.P.D. and Rothbard, A.B.S.D.: Racial disparities in antipsychotic prescription patterns for patients with schizophrenia. American Journal of Psychiatry, 2002; 159(4): 567-572.

15. Bloche, M.G.: Race and discretion in American medicine. Yale Journal of Health Policy, Law and Ethnics, 2001; 1:95-131.

16. Del Paggio, D.: Clinical and Economic Outcomes Associated with Olanzapine for the Treatment of Psychotic Symptoms in a County Mental Health Population. Clinical Therapeutics, 2002; 24:5, 1-16.

17. Smedley, B.D., Stith, A.Y. and Nelson, A.R., Eds. Unequal Treatment: Confronting Racial and Ethnic Disparities in Health Care, 2002. Washington, D.C.: National Academy Press.

18. U.S. Public Health Service Syphilis Study at Tuskegee Timeline, Center for Disease Control and Prevention, www.cdc.gov/tuskegee/timeline.htm

19. Freimuth, V.S., Quinn, S.C., Thomas, S.B., Cole, G., Zook,E., Duncan, T.: Social Science and Medicine 52, 797-808. 2001.

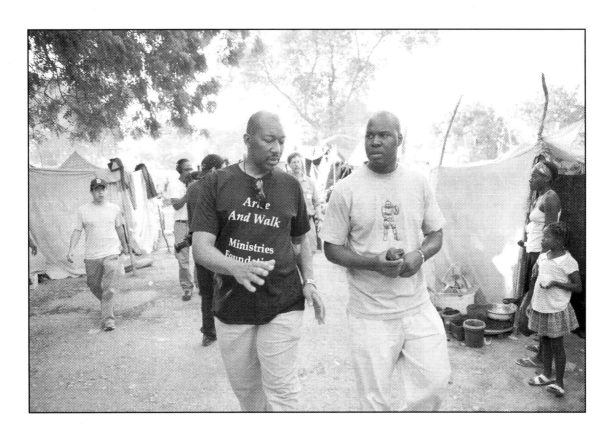

Dr. Bailey talks to leader of a refugee camp about its residents in Port-Au-Prince, Haiti.
Photo by Janet Caldwell, Meharry Medical College.

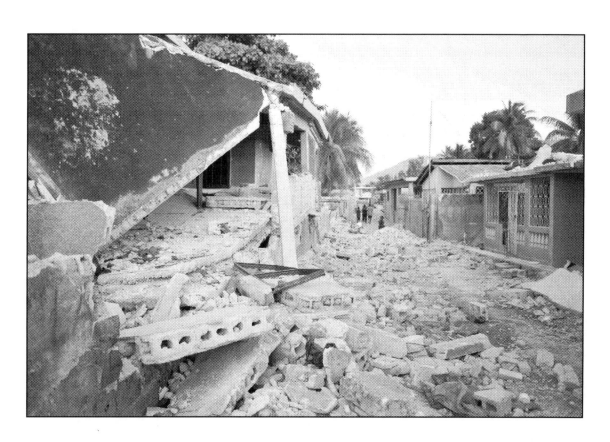

A view of the devastation in Port-Au-Prince, Haiti where Dr. Bailey and other doctors tried to bring comfort to grief-stricken earthquake victims. Photo by Janet Caldwell, Meharry Medical College.

CHAPTER 5
Gun Violence and Its Impact on Health Care

The debate between gun violence and mental illness collided on Dec. 13, 2012 when authorities said Adam Lanza walked into the Sandy Hook Elementary School in Newtown, Conn., shot and killed 20 school children and six adults in one of the most violent school shootings in U.S. history. As news spread of the horror of the murdered schoolchildren, activists, health care professionals and politicians started to speak out about what should be done to prevent a repeated event. Mental health officials have long advocated for better access to treatment for their patients. While it is debatable what role mental illness played in the Sandy Hook school shooting, many agree that a mental health component should be prominent in suggestions on how to stop such violence in the future.

Working with public and private sectors, the National Medical Association believes there are three steps that can be taken to make a significant impact to prevent such school shootings and other gun violence incidents in our country (3).

The first step is prevention. Physicians are trained to detect subtle signs of fragile and potentially violent thinking. States must support mental health programs with words, actions and resources.

The second step is risk management. Our country needs more restricted limits on gun ownership and a ban on the sale of assault weapons as a first step. Background checks could discourage some criminals and mentally ill people from purchasing guns. While we recognize that there is a profitable black market and other dealers outside of gun shows, this action is just one in a combination of actions that should be utilized to slow the spread of some of the more dangerous weapons.

The third step is education. We should move to educate our society about the violence in video games and the easy access to these games by children and teenagers. This access gives impressionable young people that this level of violence is the norm, not the exception. This is an area that needs additional research and a response to how to make this type of entertainment more responsible. We cannot afford to ignore this issue.

The NMA and Gun Violence Prevention

African-American doctors are acutely aware of the role gun violence plays in American society. While treating many of the patients in poor and urban areas, NMA members have long seen the impact of gun violence on health care. Chicago received significant media coverage last year for its homicide rate, the vast majority due to gun violence. In 2012, Chicago's homicide numbers topped the 500 mark for the first time since 2008 (1). Law enforcement officials said the deadly mix of gang activity coupled with the proliferation of guns accounted for the increase. The NMA is encouraged by the Obama Administration's Gun Violence Prevention Task Force recommendations that directly affect health care professionals and their patients (2). Those recommendations include the following:

- Directing the Centers for Disease Control and Prevention (CDC) to resume public health research on gun violence;
- Clarifying mental health benefits under the Affordable Care Act (ACA);
- Reminding doctors that the ACA does not prohibit asking their patients about guns in their homes;
- Releasing a letter to state health officials clarifying the scope of mental health services that Medicaid plans must cover;
- Finalizing regulations clarifying essential health benefits and parity requirements within ACA exchanges;
- Committing to finalizing mental health parity regulations and launching a national dialogue on mental health (3).

The nation's leading organization of psychiatrists, the American Psychiatric Association, has announced its support for President Obama's gun initiatives as well. Dr. Dilip Jeste,

President of the APA, said there should be an effort to resolve this dilemma with facts and not a pitchfork and torch mentality against those who suffer from mental illness.

"Research shows that 96 percent of people with serious mental illnesses never act violently," Dr. Jeste said in a recent APA statement about gun violence. "A vast majority of violent crimes are not committed by people with mental disorders... Research also shows that people with mental illnesses who engage in regular treatment are much less likely to commit violent acts than those who need, but are not engaged in, appropriate mental health care. And yet, in spite of evidence for effectiveness of mental health treatment, funding for public mental health services has plunged in the last few years."

Dr. Jeste and the APA support the Obama administration's plans to finalize rules governing mental health parity under the Mental Health Parity Act, the Affordable Care Act, and Medicaid. Like the NMA, the APA sees the long-term benefit of investing in mental health programs and how that will benefit the country as a whole.

"Such an outcome will be the best tribute to the memory of the innocent children and brave school staff that lost their lives a month ago," Jeste said.

Scapegoating the Mentally Ill

While recognizing the importance of mental illness treatment when it comes to guns and gun violence, the mentally ill should not be made the scapegoat of events like Sandy Hook or gun violence in general. The reality is that the mentally ill in this country are more likely to be victims of violent crime than the perpetrators (5). According to the Treatment Advocacy Center, an estimated one percent of individuals with untreated severe mental illness commit acts of violence while 25 percent of violence victims are mentally ill. According to a Feb. 27, 2012 article on MedPage Today, the mentally ill are 28.6 percent more likely to be victims of violent crime than those without a disability (6).

Many mental health professionals have expressed concern about the potential risks to patient confidentiality, increased stigma and barriers to persons needing mental health evaluation. The organization is committed to working with the federal, state and local agencies in developing the protocols for implementation. Health care professionals must be at the table from the beginning and seen as invaluable partners in addressing gun violence (3).

The NMA is uniquely prepared to partner with others and lead aspects of this national gun-control initiative. As the nation's leading African-American psychiatrists, trauma surgeons, emergency room, and primary care physicians, NMA members are on the front lines every day trying our best to repair the damage done by an unconscionable amount of violence to victims and their families – both physically and mentally.

Mental Health and Criminal Justice

Proper treatment of those suffering from mental illness in the criminal justice system has long been a concern since the deinstitutionalization of psychiatric hospitals across the country beginning in the late 1960s. A major concern of health care professionals is that those with mental illness issues caught up in the criminal justice system are not getting the care they need. That drives up recidivism rates and endangers not only the general public but the person suffering from mental illness as well. An Aug. 30, 2009 article in the Toledo Blade focused on a study from the Journal of Psychiatric Services that jail administrators in the United States should expect that from 11 percent to 18.9 percent of male prisoners and from 21.7 percent to 42.1 percent of female prisoners have some form of serious mental illness. "Jails are used in lieu of mental health hospitals," Toledo Municipal Court Judge Timothy Kuhlman was quoted in the article. "And they're not the best place to do that … and that's unfortunate." (7)

The challenge of confronting mental illness in the criminal justice system becomes more complicated when race is involved. Mental health issues are still taboo for many in the African-American community. A 1996 article, the Mental Health Association reported that 63 percent of blacks saw depression as a personal weakness and only 31 percent saw it as a health issue (8). That could explain in part the disproportionate rate of African-Americans in prison. A 2007 article by Diversity Inc. magazine noted that one in every 15 African-American men in the United States was incarcerated. That number increased to one in every nine for black men ages 20 to 34. That is compared to one in 106 white men (9).

The False Comfort of Labels

Many mental health professionals will agree that increased services in this field are sorely needed but it's not a cure all. There are many factors that go into a person attempting and succeeding to kill a mass of people. Focusing only on the mentally ill is a quick fix to something that is multilayered and has a multipronged solution. Without such a solution, which includes tackling the difficult political issue of gun proliferation, the problem will likely remain elusive. The National Rifle Association has put a stronger focus on mental health and violent video games as a stronger contributor to gun violence than the proliferation of guns. That's not surprising. As an organization that supports unabridged gun rights, that should be expected. But it should be placed in its proper context.

How do we prevent an incident like what occurred as Sandy Hook Elementary School from happening again? All options should be on the table. Trying to determine if Adam Lanza's alleged autism or Asperger's syndrome was the sole cause of his actions is simply an inefficient way to answer that question. What drives a person to shoot six-year-old children multiple times – as well as seek out the means to carry out such carnage – is complicated and challenging. Simplifying it by labeling Lanza with some mental condition and settling for that as the answer is a mistake. Care for the mentally ill is one part of the equation, but so is the means of committing the crime.

References

1. Babwin, D. Chicago Homicide Rate 2013 Already at 40 Before End of January, Huff Post Chicago/ Associated Press, Jan. 28, 2013. www.huffingtonpost.com/2013/01/28/chicago-homicide-rate-201_n_2569472.html

2. C-SPAN. White House Anti-Gun Violence Task Force Proposals, Jan. 16, 2013. http://www.c-spanvideo.org/program/AntiGu

3. Welborn C. National Medical Association Commends President Obama's Actions on Gun Violence but Issues Cautions and Concerns. Press Release, Jan. 17, 2013. http://www.nmanet.org/images/pdfs/jan17-nma_press_release.pdf

4. Jeste, D. APA President Dilip MD Video Message No. 4 – Mental Health and Gun Violence, January, 2013. www.psych.org/.../Jeste-Video-Talk-Gun-Violence-Jan-13.pdf

5. Treatment Advocacy Center Blog. New Study: Mentally Ill Are Often Targets of Violence, Treatment Advocacy Center, Arlington, Va. http://www.treatmentadvocacycenter.org/about-us/our-blog/69-no-state/2030-new-study-mentally-ill-are-often-targets-of-violence

6. Phend C. Mentally Ill Often Targets of Violence. MedPage Today, Feb. 27, 2012. http://www.medpagetoday.com/Psychiatry/GeneralPsychiatry/31383

7. Satgija N. Toledo Jails Facing Growing Number of the Mentally Ill: Inmate Influx Is Attribute to Fewer Hospitals. Toledo Blade, Aug. 30, 2009.

8. Mental Health: Culture, Race, and Ethnic Supplement-1999 U.S. Surgeon General's Report on Mental Health, Mental Health America.

9. Hannah, D. 1 in 100 Now Behind Bars; Numbers for Blacks and Latinos Bleak. Diversity Inc. magazine. http://diversityinc.com/public/3148print.cfm

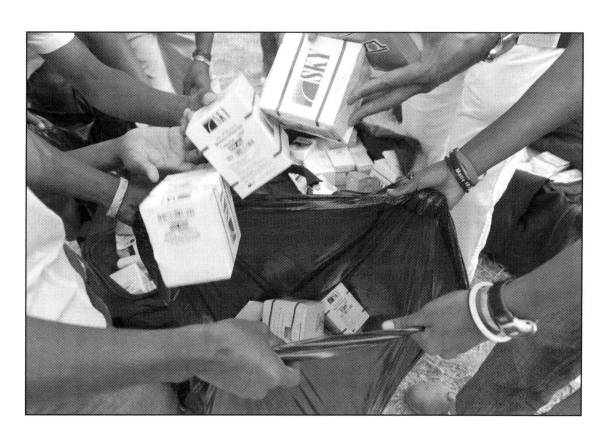

(4571) Doctors and health care workers brought boxes and medicine and other medical supplies to Haiti to help residents. Photo by Janet Caldwell, Meharry Medical College.

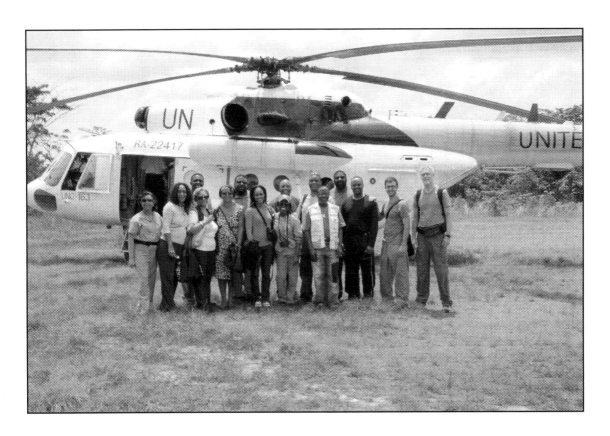

Physicians and supporters of the National Medical Association prepare to take a United Nations helicopter from Monrovia, Liberia to Jackson F. Doe Memorial Regional Referral Hospital in Tappita, Liberia.

CHAPTER 6
Facts and Myths Surrounding African-Americans and ADHD

Coauthor: Dion LaPoint Owens, MD

Tackling the myths and misinformation surrounding Attention-Deficit/Hyperactivity Disorder (ADHD) in the African-American community can be one of the most difficult issues in mental health. There is a lot of conflicting information regarding the diagnosis and treatment of African-Americans. This chapter aims to discuss some of the misconceptions and give readers more information about what to look for and what questions to ask.

The incidence of ADHD is probably similar in African-Americans and whites. However, fewer African-Americans than whites are diagnosed and treated for ADHD. That reality alone flies in the face of some perceptions in many black communities. Reasons for this disparity have not been fully clarified and are most likely complex and numerous. Some barriers to treatment are driven by the beliefs of patients and their families while others are due to limitations in the health care system. Patient-driven obstacles to care include inadequate knowledge of symptoms, treatment, and consequences of untreated ADHD including fear of over-diagnosis and misdiagnosis.

A survey conducted to explore cultural differences between African-American and white respondents about ADHD found that African-Americans were more likely than whites to be unfamiliar with ADHD. In addition, African-Americans felt that they were diagnosed with ADHD more often than whites and teachers blamed ADHD for learning or behavioral problems more often in African-Americans.

Health system barriers include a lack of culturally competent health care providers, stereotyping/biases, and failure of the clinician to evaluate the child in multiple settings before diagnosis. Strategies to overcome these challenges include increased dissemination of ADHD information through community events, improved training of clinicians in cultural competence, and open communication among parents, clinicians, and school personnel.

Basics of ADHD

Attention-Deficit/Hyperactivity Disorder is a neurological disorder characterized by hyperactivity, impulsivity, and inattention. The causes of ADHD are thought to involve genetic factors and dysfunction of the complex substances in the brain (1). Co-occurring psychiatric diseases such as conduct disorder, oppositional defiant disorder, depression, anxiety, learning disabilities, and alcohol or drug addiction are often noted in patients with ADHD.

The primary goals of therapy for ADHD are to decrease disruptive behaviors, enhance academic performance, improve relationships with family and peers, improve self-esteem, and promote independence. The prevalence of ADHD in African-Americans is most likely similar to that among the general population; however, fewer African-Americans are diagnosed and treated for ADHD (2-6). The reasons for this phenomenon have not been fully explained. However, the challenges related to insufficient diagnosis and treatment of ADHD in this population must not be oversimplified because a myriad of factors most likely contribute to the complexity of this issue.

To increase awareness among health care providers regarding the special needs of this patient population, barriers to the diagnosis and treatment of ADHD in African-Americans must be explored. This chapter will identify some potential obstacles to the care of ADHD in African-Americans and offers suggestions for intervention that are targeted to patients and their families and to health care providers (7). The success of ADHD treatment requires that these hurdles be overcome. The first crucial step involves increasing awareness among parents and other caregivers and members of the medical community.

Patient-Driven Obstacles to ADHD Care

Similar to parents from other ethnic backgrounds, many African-American parents are not well informed about the symptoms and treatment of ADHD. However, results of recent studies suggest that African-American parents may be even more uninformed about the causes and treatment of ADHD than are parents from other ethnic or racial backgrounds (8-10). One study that sought to identify differences in ADHD knowledge between 224 African-American parents and 262 white parents reported that only 69 percent of African-Americans had ever heard about ADHD compared with 95 percent of white parents .Only 36 percent of African-Americans knew "a lot," "some," or "a little" about ADHD compared with 70 percent of white parents. (8) In addition, African-American parents reported that only 18 percent received information about ADHD from their physician compared with 29 percent of white parents (8). Of note, this study found the effects of ethnicity on ADHD familiarity were independent of other covariates, such as socioeconomic status. The reasons for this disparity are unknown.

African-American families may not attribute the symptoms of ADHD to the disease itself and are less aware about the possible causes of ADHD than white families. For example, sugar intake has been reported as a common explanation for the symptoms of ADHD among members of the African-American community. (11, 8) One study reported that twice as many African-Americans parents as white parents of children with learning disabilities felt that ADHD was caused by excessive sugar consumption, and that only 10 percent of African-American parents were certain that sugar did not cause ADHD compared with 37 percent of white parents.

Furthermore, compared with 91 percent of white parents, only 75 percent of African-American caregivers thought that ADHD had genetic causes.

Medical labels such as ADHD, ADD, attention deficit, or hyperactivity were used by only 25 percent of African-Americans to describe their child's condition compared with 62 percent of white parents (8). The lack of knowledge about ADHD among the African-American community has been described as a "vicious cycle" that may be caused when members of this community seek medical advice from other individuals within their own ethnic background who are equally uninformed about ADHD (8). Data shows that African-American parents are less likely than white parents to associate the demands of school with the exacerbation of ADHD symptoms.

In addition, African-American parents of children with ADHD were less likely than white parents to request pharmacological treatment or school interventions and were less likely to mention emotion-based outcomes such as conduct disturbance. A potential disconnect between African-American parents and the school system was suggested based on the fact that African-American parents expressed fewer worries about ADHD-related school problems and fewer preferences for school intervention. In addition, fewer African-

American parents than white parents acknowledged the role of the school system in the identification of ADHD in their children. Investigators hypothesized that lower rates of parental awareness about school problems may result in lower rates of medical treatment.

African-American parents may feel more uneasy than white parents about treating their children with medications. Medical research demonstrated that significantly more African-American parents (63 percent) than white parents (29 percent) thought that counseling was the best treatment for ADHD, whereas medication was preferred over counseling in 59 percent of white parents and in 36 percent of African-American parents. Furthermore, more African-American parents than white parents felt that use of stimulants would lead to drug abuse and adverse effects. For some African-Americans, socioeconomic barriers include the lack of medical insurance, high costs of mental health care and prescription drugs. Because of this, access to behavior modification programs, school consultation, parent management training, or other specialized services is often limited (12). It is important to note that no federally funded special education programs are designed for children with ADHD. (13) Therefore, students who rely on these government services remain underserved.

Additional barriers to the treatment and diagnosis of ADHD must be considered. For example, many parents fear the perceived social stigma of an ADHD diagnosis, and some fear over-diagnosis and misdiagnosis. Pressure from family and friends to refrain from seeking treatment, fear of jeopardizing future employment or ability to serve in the military, concern that parenting skills will be questioned, and fear of the unknown are other factors that have been described by patients and families and are thought to impact the diagnosis and treatment of ADHD (13). In the African-American population, fear of the unknown may be related in part to the consequences of the Tuskegee experiment, which caused many African-Americans to lose trust in the field of medical research (14). These feelings may cause some African-American parents to question the treatment of ADHD.

A survey conducted from May to July of 2002 explored cultural differences between African-American and white respondents to identify barriers to the treatment of ADHD. The data demonstrated some important differences between ethnic groups with regard to attitudes and perceptions about ADHD (7). For example, the stigma of ADHD and lack of information about ADHD were found to be significant barriers to treatment among African-Americans.

African-American respondents were more likely than white respondents to say that they were "not at all familiar" with ADHD (7). African-American respondents were less likely than white respondents to believe that ADHD is a "very serious" condition. Compared with white respondents, African-American respondents were much more likely to believe that minority children were more apt to be told that they have ADHD and were more often misdiagnosed than were white respondents. Together with findings from other studies, data suggests that the need is great for increased awareness and information among members of the African-American community about ADHD, including the symptoms that might be observed, the consequences of untreated disease, and indications that a health care professional should be contacted.

Health System Barriers and Other Obstacles

A substantial number of obstacles to the successful diagnosis and treatment of ADHD overall are related to limitations in the diagnosis and treatment of ADHD in African-American patients. Some of these barriers may be easier to remove than others. For example, one hurdle relates to the influence of race or ethnicity alone on the diagnosis of ADHD in African-Americans (16). During the clinician-patient encounter, negative social stereotypes are known to shape behaviors and influence decisions made by health care providers (17). Race or ethnicity is known to influence the medical care provided for other conditions, as seen in referrals for cardiac procedures, analgesic prescribing, and treatment of cancer or depression (18-23). Thus, patients with ADHD are likely to be affected by this disparity as well.

Perhaps one of the most important aspects of the disparity in diagnosis and treatment among races involves important cultural differences that exist among persons of diverse ethnic backgrounds with regard to attitudes and beliefs about illness, choice of care, access to care, degree of trust toward authority figures or institutions, and tolerance for certain behaviors. Often, the quality of health care is compromised when health care providers are insensitive to cultural differences among their patients (23). Clinicians may consider using ethnically sensitive, structured parent questionnaires or rating scales in the diagnosis of ADHD in African-American children. The use of culturally sensitive diagnostic tools may assist investigators in uncovering important aspects about ADHD that may be unique to the African-American population.

Ethnic or cultural sensitivity involves a broad understanding of cultural concepts and issues and a great awareness of cultural differences in responses and care needs of patients. The need to increase cultural competence in health care is described in detail in Healthy People 2020, which is a statement of national health objectives that was designed to identify the most significant preventable threats to health and to establish national goals to reduce these threats (26, 23).

Conscious and unconscious bias or prejudice can cause the cross-cultural diagnosis of ADHD to be challenging. A commonly held misperception is that African-American children are normally more active than their peers from other ethnic backgrounds. A large study reported that African-American children were rated by teachers as more hyperactive than expected, except in schools that were located in white, middle-class neighborhoods, where the frequency of hyperactivity was consistent across all ethnic groups (16). Therefore, differences in activity level may be related to socioeconomic status rather than ethnicity.

Need for More Minority Health Care Providers

Another obstacle preventing optimal care for ADHD in African-American children is a lack of culturally competent health care providers and teachers. One case report described an African-American mother who experienced feelings of intercultural mistrust after it was suggested by a white teacher that her son should be evaluated for ADHD. This mother expressed that the real problem was "an inexperienced white teacher who wants to drug children into compliance." However, after receiving education about ADHD and directly observing her son during the school session, this parent acknowledged the importance of diagnosis and the usefulness of medical and behavioral treatments. Hence, recruiting the parent as an ally can help the clinician to pave the way to acceptance and trust.

Other health system barriers include a greater tendency of clinicians to solely rely on parent input rather than teacher input when diagnosing ADHD, as well as poor communication between medical professionals and those who implement and monitor treatment in schools. These factors may inhibit the objective diagnosis of ADHD in some children or may limit the ability of the clinician to manage pharmacological treatment.

Strategies for Intervention

To improve outcomes in African-Americans with ADHD, a number of strategies are suggested. They target at increasing awareness about ADHD, decreasing stigmatization, and teaching the benefits of ADHD treatment. For example, health care and educational services must be integrated. Patients and their families should have greater access to culturally sensitive materials or programs that educate families about the symptoms of ADHD and teach them how treatment can improve behaviors. Educating patients allows them the opportunity to become partners in their own care and increases the likelihood that patients will cooperate as much as possible. Often, if the patient does not understand the importance of treatment or follow-up care, medical care becomes compromised. Disease management requires adherence to treatment regimens and medical appointments.

Clinicians and health care providers can make substantial efforts in improving outcomes by initiating pilot programs that track the long term effectiveness of care. For example, collaborative efforts should be made among schools, primary care providers, and service agencies to monitor the symptoms of ADHD and the response to treatment. Successful disease management is contingent on cooperation and open communication among these caretakers. To alleviate issues of cross-cultural bias and mistrust, it is also of great importance that a sufficient number of minority health care providers in schools, clinics and hospitals be ensured. Thus, health care organizations must recruit and retain a diverse staff whose demographic characteristics are representative of the service area.

Health care institutions must consider ways of offering improved access to medical services and raising the level of awareness in the community. This can be accomplished in many ways. For example, information can be disseminated during community events and in churches and daycare centers to teach about ADHD, raise awareness regarding the importance of treatment, and lessen fears of stigmatization. Health fairs can be conducted to screen for ADHD. Group programs afford the opportunity for involvement of multifamily groups, which can improve the level of moral support the patient receives while undergoing treatment.

Health care providers must be diligent in their commitment to reduce or remove barriers to the proper diagnosis and treatment of ADHD in African-Americans. Efforts should be made to:

1. Increase awareness in the African-American community regarding the symptoms of ADHD and its treatment.
2. Improve cultural awareness and sensitivity toward African-American patients to reduce the challenges involved in cross-cultural diagnosis.

References

1. Rappley M. Attention deficit-hyperactivity disorder. N Engl J Med. 2005;352:165-173.
2. Rowland AS, Umbach DM, Stallone L, Naftel J, Bohlig EM, Sandler DP. Prevalence of medication

treatment for attention deficit–hyperactivity disorder among elementary school children in Johnston County, North Carolina. Am J Public Health. 2002;92:231-234.

3. Safer DJ, Zito JM. Psychotrophic medication for ADHD. Ment Retard Dev Disabil Res Rev. 1999;5:237-242.

4. Zito JM, Safer DJ, dos Reis S, Riddle MA. Racial disparity in psychotropic edications prescribed for youths with Medicaid insurance in Maryland. J Am Acad Child Adolesc Psychiatry. 1998;37:179-184.

5. Jensen PS. Epidemiologic research on ADHD: what we know and what we need to learn. Available at: www.cdc.gov/ncddd/adhd/dadabepi.htm Accessed on January 10, 2005.

6. Pastor PN, Reuben CA. Attention deficit disorder and learning disability: United States, 1997-98. National Center for Health Statistics. Vital Health Stat. 10(206). 2002.

7. Data on File, Harris Interactive.

8. Bussing R, Schoenberg NE, Perwien AR. Knowledge and information about ADHD:evidence of cultural differences among African-American and white parents. Soc Sci Med. 1998;46:919-928.

9. Mattox G. African-American youngsters inadequately treated for ADHD. Psychiatric News. 2001; 36:17.

10. Visser SN, Malone LM, Lesesne CA. Socio-demographic difference among a ational sample of African-American and white youth with attention-deficit/hyperactivity disorder. Presented at the 131st Annual Meeting of the American Public Health Association; November 17, 2003 [abstract 55745].

11. Anonymous. National Institutes of Health Consensus Development Conference Statement: diagnosis and treatment of attention-deficit/hyperactivity disorder (ADHD). JAm Acad Child Adolesc Psychiatry. 2000;39:182-193.

12. Shavers VL, Lynch CF, Burmeister LF. Knowledge of the Tuskegee study and its impact on the willingness to participate in medical research studies. J Natl Med Assoc. 2000;92:563-572.

13. Gingerich KJ, Turnock P, Litfin JK, Rosen LA. Diversity and attention deficit hyperactivity disorder. J Clin Psychol. 1998;54:415-426.

14. Geiger JH. Racial stereotyping and medicine: the need for cultural competence. Can Med Assoc J. 2001;164:1699-1700.

15. Giles WH, Anda RF, Casper ML, Esconbedo LG, Taylor HA. Race and sex differences in rates of invasive cardiac procedures in US hospitals. Data from the National Hospital Discharge Survey. Arch Intern Med. 1995;155:318-324.

16. Shiefer SE, Escarce JJ, Schulman KA. Race and sex differences in the management of coronary artery disease. Am Heart J. 2000;139:848-857.

17. Todd N, Samaroo N, Hoffman JR. Ethnicity as a risk factor for inadequate emergency department analgesia. JAMA. 1993;269:1537-1539.

18. Bach PB, Cramer LD, Warren JL, Begg CB. Racial differences in the treatment of earlystage lung cancer. N Engl J Med. 1999;341:1198-1205.

19. Young AS, Klap R, Sherbourne CD, Wells KB. The quality of care for depressive and anxiety disorders in the United States. Arch Gen Psychiatry. 2001;58:55-61.

20. US Department of Health and Human Services. Healthy People 2010. 2nd ed. Washington, DC: US Government Printing Office; 2000.

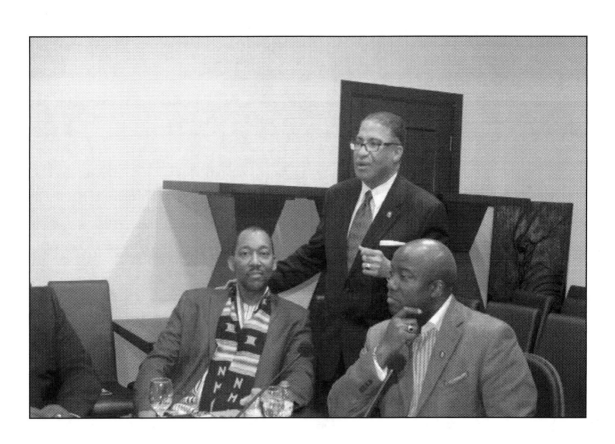

Dr. Bailey (left) and Darryl Matthews, Sr. (center), executive director of the National Medical Association, address a meeting of NMA and Liberian officials during a 2013 trip to the country.

CHAPTER 7
Major Depressive Disorder in the African-American Population

Coauthor: Holly Blackmon, BA

Major Depressive disorder (MDD) is a common and disabling psychiatric disorder in the United States that occurs across all racial and ethnic groups (1-3). It is the world's fourth leading cause of disability and the leading cause of nonfatal disease burden responsible for almost 12 percent of total years lived with disability (4). A study by Kessler using data from National Comorbidity Survey Replication found that MDD accounts for 27.2 lost work days per ill worker per year(5). This estimate includes absenteeism (work days missed) and presenteeism (poor performance on the job). Thus, the data highlight the impact that depression can have on people and society.

It is estimated that by the year 2053, nearly half the entire population will be composed of ethnic and racially diverse people (6). With this growing rate of diverse groups, clinicians and researchers will need to understand that the Eurocentric views peculiar to whites may not be relevant or adequate to address the mental health need among African-Americans and other racially diverse groups (6). All physicians, those of African-American descent and from other groups, are in need of this important information.

Rahn Kennedy Bailey, MD, DFAPA

Factors contributing to depression in African-Americans

The rate of major depression in African-Americans in the United States is considerably high. In a study by Dr. David R. Williams and colleagues that included 6,082 patients, 3,570 of whom were American blacks, the 12-month prevalence of depression in African-Americans was reported to be 5.9 percent while the lifetime prevalence rate was reported to be 10.4 percent (27-29).There are several possible factors contributing to depressed moods in African-Americans. Dr. Charlotte Brown and colleagues noted in 1996 that African-Americans have been found to report more psychosocial stressors and distress than whites, which may contribute to these high prevalence rates (29). Furthermore, the Surgeon General's landmark report in 2000 delineated specifically that factors such as lack of access to treatment, low socioeconomic status, low educational level, and low quality of treatment may present significant barriers to diagnosis and treatment of clinical depression in the African-American population.

Assessment Issues in African-Americans

The signs and symptoms of depression include depressed mood, loss of interest, loss of pleasure, significant weight or appetite change, sleep disturbance, psychomotor disturbance, fatigue/ loss of energy, feeling of worthlessness or guilt, impaired concentration, and thoughts of death or suicide. Due to numerous possibilities of the presentation of depression, diagnosis can be difficult. When considering severity of depression, a study by Williams and colleagues showed that when compared to Caucasians, African-Americans were more likely to indicate that their episodes of depression were either severe or very severe and disabling (7). More than 56.6 percent of African-Americans, compared to 38.6 percent of Caucasians, reported their episodes of depression as being disabling.

Assessment issues should be considered in the African-American community. The issue of stigma can be an obstacle in the assessment and clinical treatment in African-Americans more than any other issue. Stigma influences the diagnosis or leads to misdiagnosis, affects the attitudes that limit overall presentation, and causes African-Americans to go to a primary care doctor rather than a psychiatrist. These assessment issues to consider in the African-American population include the misdiagnosis of major depressive disorder, somatic symptom presentation, attitudes and beliefs towards depression, and stigma surrounding depression and where African-Americans typically seek treatment for their depression (8).

Psychiatric Misdiagnosis of African-Americans

A very sobering point is that African-American patients are more often incorrectly diagnosed than whites (9-10). Race and ethnicity have been shown to be a factor in accurate psychiatric diagnosis. One must consider that this is a likely phenomenon in part because of the subjective nature of psychiatric diagnosis. The ongoing research assesses this issue. A variety of reasons exist for such discrepancy in psychiatric diagnostic patterns. Limited resources may impair the ability of some African-American patients in receiving a quality psychiatric evaluation and assessment initially (6). Subsequently, once an evaluation has been conducted there is a risk that interpersonal bias can play a role in altering the correctness of psychiatric diagnosis (11). We are aware that there are certain strategies/tools that can be implemented in order to address these areas of concern. One is the enhancement of high-quality training of all clinicians in cultural competency. Such training has the potential to level the playing field and thereby increase the likelihood that all clinicians regardless of background will be prepared to make quality and unbiased evaluation of African-American patients for clinical depression (12).

African-American patients, as a group, are more likely to present with somatic symptoms compared with their white counterparts. Data from Robins and Reiger showed 15 percent of African-Americans displayed symptomatic symptoms compared to nine percent of whites (13).

Stigma, Attitudes and Beliefs of African-Americans towards Depression

One of the biggest impediments to the successful treatment of clinical depression is the issue of stigma. Dr. Annelle Prim, director of minority and national affairs for the American Psychiatric Association, expressed that such stigma is worse in African-Americans in part because of social factors specific to their culture (14). Several identified factors which may contribute to this problem include strongly held religious beliefs, lack of trust in the medical profession, communication barriers, and the long history of suffering in the African-American community (14). Clearly, these issues require a more active process in order to satisfactorily screen for this disorder. In 1996 the National Mental Association commissioned a national survey on clinical depression. The survey explored the barriers preventing African-Americans seeking treatment and measured overall knowledge of and attitudes towards depression. Major finding revealed that approximately 63 percent of African-Americans see depression as a "personal weakness" and 31 percent believed that depression is a health problem. Nearly 30 percent of African-Americans said they would "handle it" themselves if they were depressed, while nearly 20 percent said they would seek help for depression from friends and family. Only one-third of African-Americans said they would accept medication for depression if prescribed by a doctor. Close to two-thirds said they believed prayer and faith alone would successfully treat depression "almost all of the time" or "some of the time" (15-17).

African-Americans typically have significantly lower rates than Caucasians in seeking treatment (31). African-Americans are more likely to receive health care in outpatient hospital and emergency departments, and their mental health services are also characterized by high rates of emergency care. As a result, they are less likely to receive the continuity of treatment provided in primary care (30). African-Americans are more likely to seek treatment for their emotional distress, from primary care clinicians than from specialty mental health providers (20-21). Yet, in primary care, depression in African-Americans may be detected less often than it is in whites (10).

Access to treatment on the African American Population

Socioeconomic differences in America may play a role in the difficulties that affect African-Americans' ability to access treatment of clinical depression. African-Americans along with other racial ethnic minorities, encompass just more than half of the non-elderly uninsured- partly because they are more likely to be in low-income families whose employers are less likely to offer coverage. Twenty–one percent of the African-American population in 2005 was uninsured compared to 13 percent of the Caucasian population (18). African-Americans, along with other ethnic groups, are less likely than their Caucasian counter parts to receive standard routine care in one stable setting and are more likely to participate in low-income plans such as Medicaid. African-Americans are more likely than whites to need a regular place to receive care or to have a health care visit. They are most likely to receive health coverage from Medicare or other public providers. Barriers to quality care and access to utilization of available clinical services are possible contributors to the severity of disability associated with depression in the population.

Treatment Disparities among African Americans

African-Americans were found to be less likely than Caucasians to receive appropriate care for depression (19). They were less likely than Caucasians to receive an antidepressant when their depression was first diagnosed (27 percent vs. 44 percent); and less likely to receive selective serotonin reuptake inhibitors (SSRIs) (20-21). In a study by Miranda and colleagues, results showed that when the primary care physician makes similar choices regarding medications, African-Americans are less likely to use them (22). Most African-American primary care patients prefer counseling to medications, are less likely to find antidepressant medications acceptable for the treatment, and less likely to believe antidepressant medications are effective (23-24). In addition, African-Americans are more likely to believe that antidepressants are addictive than Caucasians (25). They may avoid or cease antidepressant treatment because of poor tolerance of certain classes of psychotropic medication (26). African-Americans tend to respond more quickly than Caucasians to antipsychotic medications and tricyclic antidepressants due to differences in drug metabolism (27).

Recommendations for improvement: Diagnosis, Treatment, Management, and Coping

As clinicians, we look for ways to improve diagnosis and to understand the role of cultural context in psychiatric diagnoses. This is critical to the accuracy of the diagnostic process. Physicians should consider stigma toward mental health illness and treatment for patients suspected to have depression. In psychiatric medicine, we have worked for years to improve the clinical treatment of depression. In this group of African-American patients, there seem to be specific strategies that are particularly helpful in this regard. One must assess the impact of stigma against mental illness. This factor alone can derail treatment, as some patients have been known to become non-compliant because of negative stigma of having a "brain illness."

In addition to asking their patients about depression, life stressors and social conflicts, physicians should ask about the relationship of these factors to the patient's somatic symptoms. Many patients will often focus on somatic concerns significantly. In doing so, the physician allows the patient's own individual keys to take priority. The ability of patients to describe their social stressors, life conflicts, and individual style of coping can be a helpful strategy in successful treatment. Maintaining a respectful, open approach in understanding a patient's style of coping with depressive symptoms, including religious beliefs, will facilitate an environment in which the patient can feel comfortable discussing their concerns.

Recommendations for Effective Major Depressive Disorder Management

Several recommendations have been postulated that in order to provide the most effective treatment for clinical depression in African-American patients, the physician must determine the patient's treatment preference (26). One should ask the patient first if they have a preference of medications or just talk therapy. If talk therapy is desired, it should be pursued. Physicians should educate patients about available treatments, including antidepressant medications, along with the onset of action and side effects (26). Patients need to be educated about the illness, treatment, and clinical depression as a disorder. Treatment adherence should be regularly checked. Clinicians should assist patients in finding strategies to overcome social or financial difficulties.

Compliance should be assiduously assessed, and the clinician should take the lead in this patient group and work actively to assist all patients in preventing the common social and financial barriers that abort the treatment process. Patients need to be educated fully about the illness and treatment options of clinical depression.

In treating depression, psychiatrists must consider some specific comorbidities (the presence of more than one disease or health condition in an individual at a given time). African-Americans have been shown for some time to consistently suffer from more episodes of obesity, hypertension and diabetes. These illnesses compounded with higher rates of chemical dependency, place patients at more risk of poor physical health and general disease. All of these concerns increase the likelihood of limited clinical functional outcomes both medically and psychiatrically.

Conclusion

Clinical depression presents a formidable burden in the African-American community. Cultural and socioeconomic factors present barriers to adequately diagnose and treat African-Americans. Metabolic differences may play a role in effective treatment response in African-Americans. Medical comorbidities may present challenges in the effective treatment of clinical depression in African-Americans. Lastly, greater participation in clinical research trials is essential for the improvement of accurate diagnosis and treatment of major depressive disorders in African-Americans.

References

1. Ronald C, Kessler RC, Berglund P. et al. Lifetime prevalence and age-ofonset distributions of DSM-1V disorders in the national cornorbidity survey eplication. *Arch* Gen *Psychiatry.* 2005; 62:593-602.

2. Demyttenaere K, Bruffaerts *R,* Posada-Villa J. et al. Prevalence, severity, and unmet need for treatment of mental disorders in the World Health Organization World Mental Health Surveys. JAMA. 2004; 291(211:2581-2590.

3. Kessler RC, Chiu WT, Demler 0, Walters EE. Prevalence, severity, and comorbidity of 12-month DSM-IV disorders in the national comorbidity survey replication. *Arch* Gen *Psychiatry.* 2005;62:617-627.

4. Ustun TB, Ayuso-Mateos JL, Chatterji S. Mothers C, Murray CJL. Global burden of depressive disorders in the year 2000. Br *J* Psychiatry. 2004; 184:386-392.

5. Kessler, RC, Akiskal HS, Ames M, et al. Prevalence and effects of mood disorders on work performance in a nationally representative sample of U.S. workers, Am !Psychiatry. 2006; 163:1561-1568.

6. Carrington CH. Clinical depression in African American women: Diagnoses, treatment, and research i Clin *Psycho!.* 2006; 62(7):779-791.

7. Williams DR, Gonzalez HM, Neighbors H, et al. Prevalence and distribution of major depressive disorder in African Americans, Caribbean Blacks, and Non-Hispanic Whites: Results from the national survey of American life. Arch *Gen Psychiatry.* 2007; 64:305-315.

8. US Department of Health and Human Services. Mental Health: Culture, Race, and Ethnicity—a Supplement to Mental Health: A Report of the Surgeon General. Rockville, MD; 2001.

9. Strakowski SM, Hawkins JM, Keck PE *Jr.* The effects of race and information variance on disagreement between psychiatric emergency service and research diagnoses in first-episode psychosis. *J* Clin Psychiatry. 1997;58(101:457-463.

10. Borowsky S. Rubenstein L, Meredith L, Camp P, Jackson-Triche M, Wells K. Who is at risk of nondetection of mental health problems in primary care? J Gen Intern Med. 2000; 15(6):381-388.

11. Adebimpe VR. Overview: White norms in psychiatric diagnosis of black American patients.Ami *Psychiatry.* 1981; 138:279-285.

12. Quimby E. Ethnography's role in assisting mental health research and clinical practice. J din Psycho!. 2006; 62:859-879.

13. Kirp DL. What school choice really means. *Atlantic* Monthly. 1993; 38-42.

14. Moran M. et al. Culture, history can keep blacks from getting depression treatment. Psychiatry *News.* 2004; 39:11-12.

15. National Mental Health Association. Depression and African Americans (facisheet). Alexandria, VA; 2000.

16. Mental Health Association in New Jersey Inc African American Outreach (African American factsheet). Verona, NJ; 2001.

17. Coridan C, et al. Meeting the Challenge: Ending Treatment Disparities for Women of Color. National Mental Health Association. Alexandria, VA; 2001.

18. The Henry *J* Kaiser Family Foundation. Key Facts: Race, Ethnicity and Medical Care; 2007. Publication No.: 6069-02

19. Kessler RC, McGonagle, KA, Zhao 5, et al. Lifetime and 12-month prevalence of *DSM-111-R* psychiatric disorders in the United States: Results from the National Comorbidity Survey. Arch Gen Psychiatry. 1994; 51:8-19.

20. Cooper-Patrick I., Gallo JJ, Gonzales JJ, Vu HT, Powe NR, Nelson C, Ford DE. Race, Gender, and Partnership in the Patient-Physician Relationship. *JAMA*. 1999;282:583-589,

21. Snowden LR, Pingitore D. Frequency and scope of mental health service delivery to African Americans in primary care. Ment Health Serv *Res*. 2002; 4:123-130.

22. Miranda J, Cooper L. Disparities in care for depression among primary care patients. J Gen *Intern* Med. 2004; 19:120-126.

23. Brody DS, Khaliq A. Thompson T. Patients' perspectives on the management of emotional distress in primary care settings. J Gen Intern Med. 1997; 12(7):403-406.

24. Dwight-Johnson M, Sherbourne C. Liao D, Wells K. Treatment preferences among depressed primary care patients. J Gen Intern Med. 2000; 15(8):527-534.

25. Cooper LA, Gonzales *JJ,* Gallo JJ, et al. The acceptability of treatment for depression among African-American, Hispanic, and White primary care patients. Med Care. 2003; 41:479-89.

26. Dos AK, Olfson M, McCurtis HL, Weissman MM. Depression in African Americans: Breaking barriers to detection and treatment: Community- based studies tend to ignore high-risk groups of African Americans. *J* Earn Practice. 2006;55(1):30-39

27. Bradford LD. CYP2D6 allele frequency in European Caucasians, Asians, Africans and their descendents. Pharmacogenomics. 2002; 3:229-243.

28. Williams DR, et al. Arch Gen Psychiatry. March 2007, 64: 305-315.

29. Brown C, et al. J of Affect Disord 41 (1996) 181-191.

30. Mental Health: Culture, Race, and Ethnicity, 2001. A Supplement to Mental Health: A Report of the Surgeon General, 2000.

31. Mental Health: Culture, Race, and Ethnicity, 2001. A Supplement to Mental Health: A Report of the Surgeon General, 2000: pg. 57.

32. Sue, S., Fujino, DC, Hu, L, Takeuchi, DT, Zane, N (1991). Community mental health services for ethnic minority groups: A test of the cultural responsiveness hypothesis. Journal of Consulting and Clinical Psychology, 59 (4), 533-540.

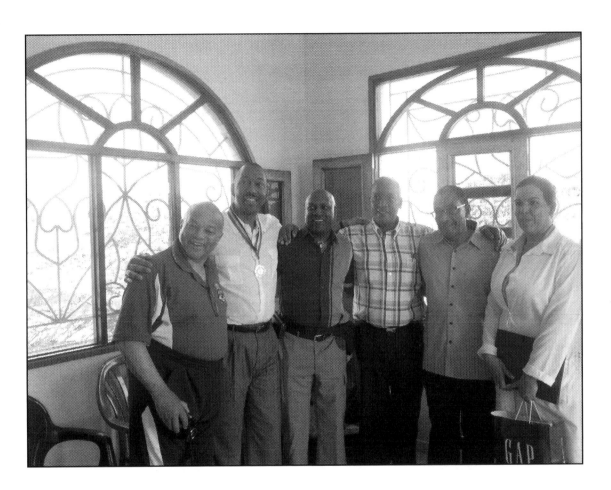

A National Medical Association delegation made a government-approved professional exchange to Cuba in February, 2013. Part of the delegation included Dr. Richard Butcher, NMA president 1992 (far left); Dr. Rahn Kennedy Bailey (second from left); Dr. Winston Price, NMA president 2004 (third from left); and Dr. Rodney Hood, NMA president 2000 (second from right).

CHAPTER 8

Atypical Antipsychotic Medicines: A Review for African-American Physicians

Now there were 12 new-generation atypical psychiatric medications available. As these new treatments have become more common, they have grown to account for a significant percentage of all psychiatric medications prescribed. This is because of their efficacy in the treatment of several psychiatric disorders, ease of administration, and absence of the well-known extrapyramidal adverse effects long-attributed to the standard dopamine blocking anti-psychotic medications. As these medications have become treatments of choice, we have discovered additional information about their respective side effects. Issues such as bone marrow suppression, endocrine abnormalities, and most recently, cardiac arrhythmias have produced concern. This chapter will address all in an attempt to inform the primary care physician of the most prominent and clinically relevant adverse effects of these agents. A particular focus will address the increasing concern that these new medications can produce hyperglycemia and diabetes mellitus.

After the introduction of Clozapine in 1989, the psychiatric marketplace has added multiple new agents effective in the treatment of psychosis, depression, anxiety and mood labiality. These new agents include Risperidone (1993), Olanzapine (1996), Quetiapine (1997) and

Ziprasidone (2001). They are known as new-generation medications since each share the aspect of having a more diverse neuroreceptor background, which leads to a broader spectrum of clinical activity. This feature differentiates them from the more traditional psychiatric choices, all of which typically worked on "limbic-specific" dopamine type 2 (D2) receptor binding, and were effective in primarily a singular clinical domain. In addition, they share having a greater than one ratio of serotonin type 2 (5HT2A) receptor binding to D2 binding. It is this distinction, which most investigators attribute to the enhanced beneficial effects on mood seen with these agents. Recent studies have shown efficacy among these medications in the treatment of acute mania (Olanzapine and Ziprasidone) (1), as add-on therapy for mood stabilization (Risperdal) (2), and even primary unipolar depression (Olanzapine)(3).

Historically problematic side-effects of the older drug treatments have primarily been neurological in nature (4). Presently, the three main areas of concern include bone marrow suppression, endocrine abnormalities such as obesity, hyperglycemia, and hyperprolactinemia, and cardiac arrhythmia (5). However, with the advent of these newer treatments, there has developed a significant focus on a different array of adverse effects. This typically led to the standard short-term problem with extra-pyramidal effects such as akathisia, dystonia and pseudo Parkinsonism, and the eventual, long-term movement disorder, tardive dyskinesia. Over the past several years, many studies have been published detailing these untoward effects and their relevance in clinical practice (6, 11, 13, 16, 17). Data with a primary focus on the pertinent concerns for the African-American primary care physician will be reviewed in this chapter.

Bone Marrow Suppression

When Clozaril became commercially available in the U.S. a decade ago, it quickly became a mixed blessing for psychiatrists and patients. Although initially hailed as a possible panacea for patients with chronic mental illness because it had been so effective in Europe since 1970, bone marrow suppression immediately led to significant concern. Specifically, the agranulocytosis that is documented to affect 1-2 percent of all patients on this treatment has limited the overall use of this agent (6). Patients can require as much as weekly checks of their serum levels to monitor for decreasing white blood cell counts (WBC). For those whose WBC count decline to below 3,000/mm, it is recommended that the use of this medication be discontinued (7).

At this point, Clozapine is the only new-generation agent indicated as a causative agent in producing bone marrow suppression (8). Cautious use of the medication is warranted due to the seriousness of this side effect. Clozapine therapy is recommended after two fairly long-term, if not exhaustive, failures with other less risky anti-psychotic medications (9). This adverse effect is a matter of concern for severely mentally ill patients, as Clozapine is the only anti-psychotic medication of any type to have been shown to be over 50 percent effective in the treatment of refractory patients when compared to Chlorpromazine (7). Those treatment refractory patients (TRS) have the same risk as well. The inability to use Clozaril openly, has most likely been a greater disadvantage to the African-American TRS patient population overall (10, 11).

Endocrine Side Effects

Endocrine abnormalities have a long history of being associated with psychiatric treatment (12). There are a variety of articles in the psychiatric literature documenting a correlation between chronic mental illness and the development of diabetes mellitus (13, 14). There is information available which documents that diabetes had developed in psychiatric patients well before the introduction of the first antipsychotic medication Chlorpromazine (Thorazine)(14). That agent became commercially available in the 1950s (15). The older antipsychotic agents such as Chlorpromazine, Haloperidol and Fluphenazine have long been reported to produce endocrine adverse effects such as impotence, amenorrhea, galactorrhea and gynecomastia (16). Now though, the new generation agents have been readily identified with a variety of the same types of endocrine clinical effects. Weight gain/ obesity, hyperglycemia and hyperprolactinemia have been most significantly studied (16).

Although all atypical medications are likely to lead to more weight gain than the older typical agents, the two atypical agents most often identified with weight gain are Clozapine and Olanzapine. Quetiapine can cause weight gain, as these are the three most antihistaminic selections of this group. Antihistaminic effects can lead to frequent sedation, and to increase appetite/weight gain among all patients. There are now many studies that have reported different proportions of weight gain in patients receiving the various medications in this group (13, 17). However, it is important to be aware that practically all of the well-structured studies in this area reveal some degree of weight gain across all of these agents (18). The most significant weight gains occur with the use of Clozapine (17).

When discussing weight gain issues, there are several important points to consider. First, one study showed that there are weight changes across the full spectrum – from significant gains to weight loss in some cases (19). There is now data that supports a biochemical alternation may be at the root cause of this well-identified weight gain by the medication in this class (20, 21). It has been reported that a change in the preference for oxidizing carbohydrates, rather than fats, may be causal factor in the increased carbohydrate craving often seen after the administration of these agents (20). This could be indicative of the periodic weight gain that can occur.

Although the general contemporary discussion most often focuses on large amounts of weight gain, there is evidence of some weight loss, or certainly weight neutrality, with particular atypical agents (22). Yet, even in the case of notable weight gain, there are now good recommendations of how to respond to these changes. A recent UCLA study reported key success in decreasing much of the medication induced weight gain via a variety of pharmacological and behavioral interventions (23). Most particularly, strategies such as recording weight regularly in all physician offices, educational programs geared to inform patients about their food selection process, and actively discussing how to manage the entire dietary process. These discussions should become a fundamental component of the routine medical management of all patients with chronic, severe and persistent mental illness (23).

All of the medicines evaluated exhibited an alteration in their documented weight gain except Clozaril (17). Nguyen and Maguire at the University of California Irvine, Littrell and Petty of the ProMedica Research Group in Atlanta, have published other similar work (24, 25). Importantly, this work composed of a variety of individuals including African-American patients. Each of these studies highlights several important themes for managing weight gain in persons on the newer atypical psychiatric medications. First, the weight gain prospects vary. Some patients will gain weight, while others will not. There is data that suggests that most persons, who gain, do so up to about 3–4 kilograms or approximately 10 pounds over an initial 60–90 day period (26). In addition, similar data points out that much of the total increases in a patient's weight that may occur often are restricted to the first 38–40 weeks of medication exposure (27). In fact, it has been shown in Olanzapine when compared to Haloperidol studies that the rate of weight gain slows after the first few weeks of treatment, reaching a plateau within six to nine months (27).

This information is important because it emphasizes the necessity of addressing these concerns in all high-risk patients as early as possible. There are data to support the use of alternate medications, non-amphetamines, to prevent the potential medication-induced appetite increases, which can occur and lead to excessive food intake (28). The anticholinergic/antiviral medication Amantadine (Symmetrel)(29), and the anti-ulcer treatment Nizatadine (Axid)(30), have been shown to be effective. These agents and others that can be used but have not been prospectively studied in clinical trials (Topiramate), can be effective in preventing some of the weight gain, though they are not as effective in decreasing the weight once it has been gained (28). It remains important to remember in face of all of this information, that all weight gained only occurs because of excessive calorie intake. Generally, this occurs as a result of an increase in appetite, particularly carbohydrates craving, which can lead to more food intake.

When excessive oral food intake develops into a pattern, the potential for hyperglycemia emerges (28). Prior studies have shown a clear association between this finding and schizophrenia (31). There is now a renewed interest due to the development of these novel agents (32). One report that addressed this correlation showed that the most likely agent to increase serum glucose of this group was Clozaril (33). It was shown to do so by an average of 13-15 mg/dl (33). Risperdal increased this marker by 3-4mg/dl in the study (33). Clearly, this increased risk factor for the development of diabetes mellitus in this cohort of patients creates a very real and important concern. However, none of the new generation agents, with the exception of Clozaril, increased this marker by the factor greater than 10 mg/dl (33).

The most often considered secondary complication related to the weight gain and hyperglycemia is the potential development of Type II diabetes (34). Diabetes mellitus has become a widespread chronic medical condition. It has been shown to have a prevalence rate of 7.8 percent in the U.S. general adult population (35). There are approximately 16–17 million persons in this country with the diagnosis of diabetes Type II. In fact, it is even more common in persons with mental illness, than in the general population (13, 36). It is also commonly seen in African-Americans and members of other ethnically diverse groups such as Hispanics and Native Americans (37). Predisposition of patients with chronic mental illness to diabetes actually predated the introduction of the standard anti-psychotic medications (14, 15). It is generally considered that there is a greater risk of Type II diabetes in psychiatric patients compared to the general population (38). This has led to a concern among psychiatric physicians that certain, if not all, of these newer agents should be avoided in this class of patients. Several key factors that need to be considered include family history, age (>45), history of glucose intolerance, and race (higher risk in African-Americans). In addition to the static factors mentioned, dynamic factors such as obesity, dyslipidemia, poor exercise habits and hypertension likewise are important (39). Furthermore, high fat diets and elevated serum prolactin can also play a significant role (39). The primary care physician, more likely than the psychiatrist, can best manage complications of weight gain, hyperglycemia, and diabetes mellitus.

Hyperprolactinemia is an endocrine condition that can be a cause for concern. Some individuals will experience clinical manifestation as a result of this condition. The most common such illnesses include amenorrhea, galactorrhea and gynecomastia. These side effects have been well documented in the psychiatric literature (40). This finding is seen most commonly in the medications that have the greatest degree of dopamine-2 receptor binding (41), such as Risperdal (42). While increased levels of prolactin can actually develop into a clinical side-effect that can eventually lead to aggression and hostility, the actual prolactin level is least likely to be directly associated with any clear-cut clinical symptoms among this group (40, 42).

Cardiac Arrhythmias

A third key untoward effect noted among the new generation atypical agent is cardiac arrhythmias. Notably, prolongation of the QT interval (the QT interval represents the time of ventricular repolarization) can be caused by certain psychiatric medication (43). The long used anti-psychotic Thioridazine (Mellaril) received a Federal Drug Administration "black box" warning in July 2000 due to this finding (8, 43). The atypical psychotropic medication most directly associated with this abnormality is Ziprasidone (Geodon), followed by Quetiapine (43). All of these agents displayed rates of QT prolongation that exceeded the recommended limit of 10 millisecond increases from the prior baseline values (43). These rates were higher than those of other atypical agents such as Risperidone and Olanzapine (43). In addition, they surpassed the rates of the typical antipsychotic agent Haldol (43).

Clinically speaking, the question arises, how is this concern relevant in practice? The QT interval allows for ventricular preparation for productive contraction. It is well-known that alterations in this time period can precipitate an arrhythmia. The most significant arrhythmia produced is Torsades de Pointes. This can actually lead to an atrial fibrillation, and subsequently a ventricular fibrillation. This QT interval is typically measured via a system developed by Brazett in 1921. The Brazett formula corrects for the inevitable differences in heart rate. This correction then produces a determination that is called the QTc, or corrected QT interval (44).

Many physicians have challenged the data showing that antipsychotics have been associated with cardiovascular morbidity and mortality (45). Some who have prescribed

Thioridazine on numerous occasions are quite skeptical about any real danger being present with its continued use (46). Clearly, it is an area of significant medicolegal concern. This concern is a real and important one because of the increased susceptibility that psychiatric patients have to all forms of chronic medical illness (45). It is an often overlooked fact that these patients are found to be at higher risk of several, commonly treatable, but incurable, disorders as compared to the general American population (45).

Neurological Side Effects

There is a long history of neurological side effects with the use of the older, standard antipsychotic medications. In fact, they were called neuroleptics because they could produce these neurological effects (47). Historically, we have often attributed the actual clinical efficacy of these agents to their ability to produce these effects. However, the classic short-term complications developed in these circumstances are called extrapyramidal symptoms (EPS). The typical EPS symptoms include dystonias, akathisia and Parkinsonian effects. They are believed to result from dopamine blockade in the nigrostriatal pathway (48). This process leads to imbalance of dopamine and acetycholine in this region of the brain. It is the occurrence that is believed to be the cause of neuroleptic induced EPS (48).

There is now new data that sheds a different and unique light on this issue. A recent study showed that the most important factor in the development of EPS is not just the aggregate number of receptors bound, but how tight those receptors are bound (49). Seeman and Tallerico showed that the more loosely bound agents (faster dissociation) are less likely to produce EPS. Quetiapine and Clozapine are documented to have the weakest dopamine binding (50).

Olanzapine is mid-range while Risperidone, Ziprasidone and the typicals exhibit the strongest affinity for the dopamine receptor of this class. Haloperidol would be considered to have extremely tight binding for the receptor. This is noted to have practical significance because Positron Emission Tomography (PET) data has shown that the percentage of dopamine receptors bound plays a key role in overall clinical efficacy (51). It is now known that about 65 percent binding of dopamine receptors in the basal ganglia region of the brain produce the desired relief of the key positive symptoms of psychosis (i.e. paranoia, hallucinations or delusions)(50). Yet, at 70-75 percent such binding is likely to produce endocrine side effects, and at 80 percent or above, the neurological symptoms of EPS can appear (50). Clearly, there is a direct clinical advantage in moving toward the newer agents with substantially less exposure to the worst forms of adverse effects, and some documented evidence of enhanced clinical treatment efficacy (45).

Treatment

There is a new and improved group of psychiatric medications available for the treatment of patients with chronic psychiatric illness. Although not perfect, because they do not completely eliminate or cure the dreaded debilitating aspects of these diseases, they substantially have enhanced the ability of all psychiatric physicians to manage the symptoms of these illnesses. Each of these new choices has been shown to be at least as effective as the prior best treatment, which was Haloperidol (52). Yet, collectively they have shown so much more. These agents have been shown effective in more than singular areas of psychiatric illness (52).

This so-called broad-spectrum efficacy has altered the treatment model of our most severely ill patients (52). It has also produced the potential for fewer medication combinations and less overall polypharmacy (53). Since Olanzapine and Ziprasidone have shown efficacy in treating acute mania as monotheraphy, and Risperidal as an add-on agent, the addition of these choices can limit the need for co-therapy between an older anti-psychotic and a traditional mood stabilizer. In addition, several of the newer agents have neuroreceptor involvement with anti-anxiety benefits. Olanzapine has been shown to be a gamma-amino butyric acid (GABA) agonist, similar to a standard benzodiazepine. Ziprasidone has been shown to have effects at the 5HT1A receptor (5). This effect is similar to that seen with the anti-anxiety agent Buspirone, which has more of a benefit in treating long-term, moderately severe anxiety in patients with disorders such as Generalized Anxiety Disorder (GAD). That being as compared to the more common treatment of severely acute anxiety such as is frequently seen with panic disorder.

These new generation medications have also been shown to have efficacy in treating the patient with Dementia. Quetiapine for example may have particular benefit in treating the elderly patient with Lewy Body Dementia. Quetiapine's sedating components are also now being used more routinely in treatment of the anxious geriatric patient. This may be the result of our increasing awareness of the adverse consequence of using anti-cholinergic medications in the elderly. These are the very choices that have for so long led to the fecal impaction dehydration, and decubitus ulcers, which lead to nursing home censure. Historically, we often added every anti-cholinergic medication to the traditional anti-psychotics to prevent the neurological adverse effects mentioned earlier. With the newer atypicals, those are not needed because the relative risk of EPS is low. In fact, a recent study has shown that Olanzapine can be effective in actually treating these side-effects such as Tardive Dyskinesia (TD) (54). This is a most important consideration in the elderly, because of their increased risk of TD. At this time, Risperidone is the most commonly prescribed psychotropic medication in the elderly institutionalized patient nationwide. Their overall efficacies at low doses (0.5mg–1.5 mg), tolerability, and broad use across an array of various psychotic patient presentations, have made it an effective choice in this area of patient care (55).

There are other psychiatric special populations that have shown responsiveness to atypical psychotropic medicines, as well. For example, both Olanzapine in children (55), and Risperidone (57) have been shown to successfully treat stuttering. In addition, there has been clinical research support of Olanzapine treatment of alcohol dependence disorders (58).

All of these issues and concerns may provide the backbone for the future treatment of the African–American psychiatric patient chronic mental illness.

Reference

1. Tohen MF, Sanger TM, et al. Olanzapine versus placebo in the treatment of acute mania. Olanzapine HGEH study group. American Journal of Psychiatry. 1999; 156:702-9.
2. Ghaemi SN, Sachs GS, Baldassano CF, et al. Acute treatment of Bipolar Disorder with adjunctive risperidone in outpatients. Canadian Journal of Psychiatry. 1997; 42:196-9.
3. Shelton RC, et al. The effectiveness of Olanzapine augmentation to fluoxetine for the treatment of resistant depression. American Journal of Psychiatry. 2001; 158: 131-134.
4. Casey DE. Clozapine. Neuroleptic inducing EPS and tardive dyskinesia. Psychopharmacology. 1989; 99: S47-S53.
5. Pfizer Inc. Geodon (Ziprasidone) package insert. New York, New York. 2001.
6. Atkin K, Kendall F, et al. Neutropenia and agranulocytosis in patients receiving clozapine in the UK and Ireland. British Journal of Psychiatry. 1996; 169: 483-8.
7. Kane J, Honigfeld G, et al. Clozapine for the Treatment Resistant Schizophrenic: A Double Blind Comparison with Chlorpromazine. Archives of General Psychiatry. 1988; 45: 789-796.
8. Physicians' Desk Reference, Montvale, NJ. Medical Economics Co., 2002.
9. Potkin SG, Bera R, Gulasekaram B, et al. Plasma clozapine concentrations predict clinical response in treatment-resistant schizophrenia. Journal of Clinical Psychiatry. 1994, 55 (Suppl B): 133-136.
10. Perry PJ, Miller DD, Arndt SV et al. Clopazine and norclozapine plasma concentrations and clinical response in treatment-refractory schizophrenics. American Journal of Psychiatry. 1991; 148: 231-235.
11. Glazer WM. Extrapyramidal side effects, tardive dyskinesia and the concept of atypicality. Journal of Clinical Psychiatry. 2000; 61 (Suppl 3): 16-21.

12. Mokdad AH, Bowman BA, et al: The continuing epidemics of obesity and diabetes in the U.S. Journal of American Medical Association. 2001; 286: 1195-1200.

13. Mukhergee S, Decina P et al. Diabetes Mellitus in schizophrenic patient. Comprehensive Psychiatry. 1996; 37: 68-73.

14. Lorenz WF. Sugar tolerance in dementia praecox and other mental disorders. Archives of Neurology and Psychiatry. 1922; 8: 184-196.

15. Charatan FBE, Bartlett NG. The effect of chlorpromazine ("Largactil") on glucose intolerance. Journal of Mental Science. 1955; 101: 351-353.

16. McIntyre RS, McCann SM, et al: Antipsychotic metabolic effects: weight gain, diabetes mellitus and lipid abnormalities. Canadian Journal of Psychiatry. 2001; 46: 273-281.

17. Wirshing DA, Wirshing WC, et al: Novel antipsychotics. Comparison of weight gain liabilities. Journal of Clinical Psychiatry. 1999; 60: 358-363.

18. Allison DB, Mentore JL, et al. Antipsychotic-induced weight gain: a comprehensive research synthesis. American Journal of Psychiatry. 1999; 156: 1686-1696.

19. O'Keefe C, Noordsy D, et al. Reversal of Weight Gain Associated with antipsychotic treatment. Presented at 154th APA Annual Meeting. May 5-10, 2001, New Orleans, La.

20. Berstein JG. Psychotropic drug induced weigh gain: mechanisms and management. Clinical Neuropharmacology. 1988; 11 (Suppl 1): S, 194-206.

21. Heisler LK, Chu HM, and Tecott LH: Epilepsy and obesity in serotonin 5-HT2C receptor mutant mice. Annals NY Academy of Sciences, 1998; 861: 74-78.

22. Glick ID, et al. Insulin Resistance in Olanzapine and Ziprasidone treated patients. Results of a double blind controlled six-week trial. Presented at the APA Meeting. New Orleans, La., 2000.

23. Wirshing DA. Adverse Effects of Atypical Antipsychotics. Journal of Clinical Psychiatry. 2001; 62 (Suppl 21): 7-10.

24. Littrell KH, Petty R, et al: Educational Intervention for the Management of antipsychotic related weight gain. Presented at 154th APA Annual Meeting May 5-10, 2001. New Orleans, La.

25. Nguyen CT, Ortiz T, et al. Nutritional Education in Minimizing Weight Gain associated with antipsychotic therapy. Presented at 154th APA Annual Meeting May 5-10, 2001. New Orleans, La.

26. Hummer M, Kemmler G, Kurz, M et al. Weight gain induced by clozapine. European neuropsychopharmacology, 1995; 5: 437-440.

27. Kinon, BJ, Basson BR, et al. Long-term Olanzapine treatment: weight change and weight-related health factors in schizophrenia. Journal of Clinical Psychiatry. 2001; 62: 92-100.

28. Basson BR, Kinon BJ, Taylor CC et al. Factors influencing weight change in patients with schizophrenia treatment with olanzapine versus haloperidol or risperidone. Presented at 51st Institute of Psychiatric Services; 1999, New Orleans, La.

29. Floris M, Deberdt W, et al. Effect of Amantadine on weight gain during Olanzapine treatment. European Neuropsychopharmacology. 2001; 11: 181-182.

30. Breier A, Tanaka Y, et al: Nizatidine for the Prevention of Olanzapine-Associated weight gain in schizophrenia and related disorder-A Randomized Controlled Double Blind Study. Presented at 41st New Clinical Drug Evaluation Unit (NCDEU); May 28-31, 2001. Phoenix, Ariz.

31. Allison DB, Fontaine KR, Heo M et al. The distribution of body mass index among individuals with and without schizophrenia. Journal of Clinical Psychiatry. 1999; 60: 215-220.

32. Melkersson KI, Hulting AL, Brismar KE: Elevated levels with insulin, leptin and blood lipids in Olanzapine-treated patients with schizophrenia or related psychosis. Journal of Clinical Psychiatry. 2000; 61: 742-749.

33. Henderson DC, Cagliero E, Gray C et al. Clozapine, diabetes mellitus, weight gain and lipid abnormalities: a five-year naturalistic study. Am J of Psychiatry 2000; 157: 975-981.

34. Rockwell WJK, Ellinwood EK Jr., Trader DW. Psychotropic drugs promoting weight gain: health risks and treatment implications. Southern Medical Journal. 1983; 76:1407-1412.

35. Rubin RJ, Altman WM, et al: Health Care Expenditures for people with diabetes mellitus, 1992. Journal of Clinical Endrocrology and Metabolism. 1994; 78: 809 A-F.

36. Mckee HA, D'Arcy PF, Wilson PJ: Diabetes and schizophrenia. Journal of Clinical and Hospital Pharmacy. 1986; 11: 297-9.

37. Harris MI, Flegal KM, et al: Prevalence of diabetes, impaired fasting glucose tolerance in U.S. adults: the Third National Health and Nutrition Examination Survey, 1988-1994. Diabetes Care. 1998; 21: 518-24.

38. Dixon L, Weiden P, Delahanty J et al. Prevalence and correlates of diabetes in national schizophrenia samples. Schizophrenia Bulletin. 2000; 26: 903-912.

39. Kraemer HC, Stice E, Kazdin A, et al. how to do risk factors work together? Mediators, moderators and independent overlapping and proxy risk factors. American Journal of Psychiatry. 2001, 158: 848-856.

40. Petty RG. Prolactin and antipsychotic medications: mechanism of action. Schizophrenia Research. 1999; 35 Suppl: S67-73.

41. Kapur S, Zipursky RB, et al: Relationship between dopamine D(2) occupancy, clinical response, and side effects: a double blind PET study of first-episode schizophrenia. American Journal of Psychiatry. 2000; 157: 514-20.

42. Conley RR: Risperidone side effects. J Clin Psychiatry. 2000; 61 suppl 8:20-3; discussion 24-5.

43. Pfizer Inc. Study report on Zipraside Clinical Pharmacology Protocol, Rockville, Md.: FDA Center for Drug Evaluation and Research Division of Cardio Renal Drug Products Consultation. June 14, 2000.

44. Ahnve S. Correction of the QT interval for heart rate: Review of different formulas and the use of Bazett's formula in myocardial infarction. American Heart Journal. 1985; 109: 568-574.

45. Meltzer HY. Outcome in schizophrenia: Beyond symptom reduction. Journal of Clinical Psychiatry. 1999; 60 (Suppl 3): 3-7.

46. Krakowski MI, Kurz M, Czobor P et al. Long-term high dose neuroleptic treatment: who gets it and why? Hospital Community Psychiatry. 1993; 44: 640-644.

47. Casey DE, Keepers GA: Neuroleptic side effects. Acute extrapyramidal symptoms and tardive dyskinesia. Psychopharmacology. Series 1988, 5:74-93.

48. Casey DE, Hirsh S, Weinberger DR, eds. Schizophrenia. Oxford, England: Blackwell; 1995: 546-565.

49. Kapur S. Seeman P. Does Fast Dissociation from the Dopamine D2 Receptor Explain the Action

of Atypical Antipsychotics? A New Hypothesis. American Journal of Psychiatry. 2001; 158:3. 360-69.

50. Seeman P and Tallerico T. Antipsychotic drugs which elicit little or no Parkinsonism bind more loosely than dopamine to brain D2 receptor, yet occupy high levels of these receptors. Molecular Psychiatry, 1998; 3: 123-134.

51. Kapur S, Zipursky RB, et al: Clinical and theoretical implications of 5-HT2 and D2 receptors occupancy of Clozapine, Risperidone and Olanzapine in schizophrenia. American Journal of Psychiatry. 1999; 156: 286-93.

52. Chakos M. Lieberman J, Hoffman E et al. Effectiveness of second-generation antipsychotics in patients with treatment-resistant schizophrenia: a review and meta-analysis of randomized trials. American Journal of Psychiatry. 2001; 158: 518-526.

53. Stahl S. Fiscal pharmacology of the novel antipsychotics: getting the biggest bang out of the buck. Orange County Psychiatric Society Meeting (sponsored by AstraZeneca, Jeanssen, Eli Lilly and Pfizer) January 2002, Dana Point, Calif.

54. Kinon BJ, Stauffer V, et al. Poster presented at APA 53rd Annual Institute of Psychiatric Services, October, 2001, Orlando, Fla.

55. Katz IR, Jeste DV, Mintzer JE, et al. Comparison of risperidone and placebo for psychosis and behavior disturbances associated with dementia: a randomized, double-blind trial. Risperidone Study Group. Journal of Clinical Psychiatry. 1999; 60: 107-115.

56. Lavid N. Franklin DL, Maguire GA. Management of child and adolescent stuttering with Olanzapine: three case report. Annals of Clinical Psychiatry. 1999; 11: 233-6.

57. Maguire GA, Riley GD, et al: Risperidone for the treatment of stuttering. Journal of Clinical Psychopharmacology. 2000; 20: 479-82.

58. Littrell KH, Petty RG et al: Olanzapine treatment for patients with schizophrenia and substance abuse. Journal of Substance Abuse and Treatment. 2001; 21: 217-21.

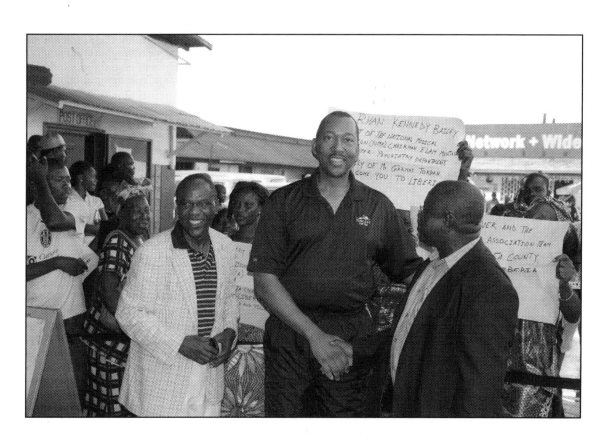

In Monrovia, Liberia, Dr. Bailey is welcomed by Dr. Francis Kateh (Medical Director of Jackson F. Doe Regional Referral Hospital) and Dr. Moses Massaquui (Director of Clinton Foundation in Liberia). Photo by Frank Glover, MD.

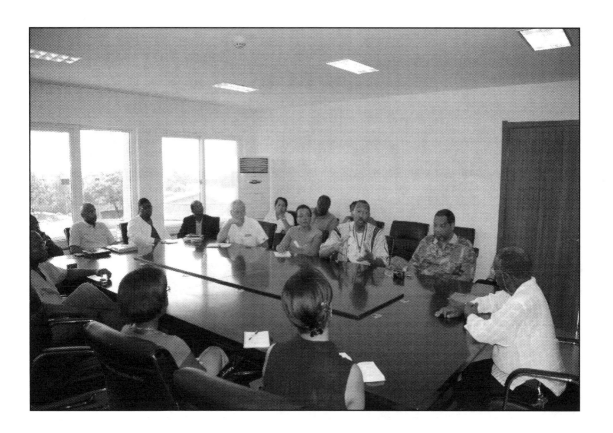

Dr. Bailey and other members of National Medical Association meet with Minister of Health and Social Welfare of Liberia, Dr. Walter T. Gwenigale.

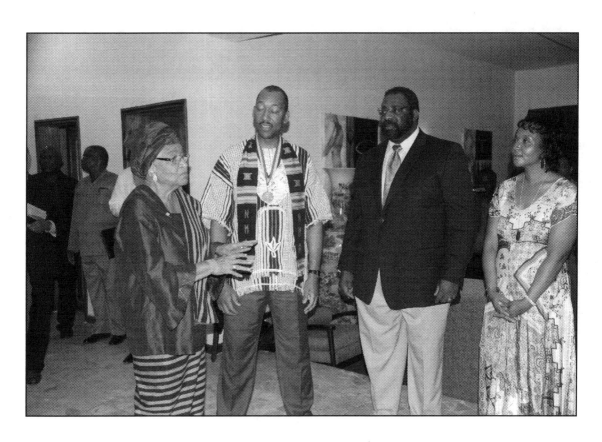

From left to right, Liberia's Honorable President Ellen Johnson Sirleaf, talks with Dr. Bailey, Dr. Frank Glover and Dr. Marsha Glover during the NMA's 2013 trip to the country.

CHAPTER 9

Health Disparities in Older Adults: An Opportunity for Reform

Author: Charles P. Mouton, MD, MS

Health disparities have been a growing focus of medical, health policy and public health organizations for the past two decades. A particular concern for those examining the risk factors, preventive strategies and outcomes related to health disparities has been the impact on race and ethnicity. Thus, a disparity means a difference to two quantities (i.e. Rate A ≠ Rate B). Several organizations have broadened this definition.

- The National Institutes of Health (NIH) defines health disparities as: "... differences in incidence, prevalence, mortality and burden of diseases or adverse health conditions that exist among specific population groups in the U.S. (1)"
- The Institute of Medicine (IOM) defines health disparities in health care as: "... racial or ethnic differences in the quality of health care that are not due to access related factors or clinical needs, preferences and appropriateness of intervention (2)."
- An the U.S. Congress in Public Law 106–525 has stated: "A population is a health disparity population if ... there is a significant disparity in the overall rate disease incidence, prevalence, morbidity, mortality or survival rates ... compared to the health status of the general population (3)."

Scholars have recognized that inequalities in health are based on observed differences such as:

- Poor die younger than rich
- Lower socioeconomic status infants have lower birth weight
- Women live longer than men
- More smokers die of lung cancer than non-smokers

However, these differences may also be thought of as inequities in health. Inequities in health are based on ethical judgments about those differences. For instance is ***it fair that:***

- Poor die younger than rich
- Lower socioeconomic status infants have lower birth weight
- Women live longer than men
- More smokers die of lung cancer than non-smokers

In this context, this chapter will exam disparities in health in older adults, particularly focusing on racial/ethnic minority populations.

Demographics of older adults, especially African-American

The importance of addressing health disparities in older adults is due to the expected growth of the older population – the demographic imperative. Adults living into older ages is continued to grow and the oldest old are showing exponential growth (4).

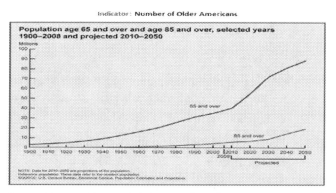

Source: United States Census Bureau, Decennial Census, Population Estimates and Projections (4). Figure 1. Changes in the age distribution of people 65 and older in the U.S. population over the last century and projected through 2050.

The older population is growing and expected to continue to grow over the next three decades. In addition, the older minority population is anticipated to grow as well with their relative percentages more that doubling in some cases (5).

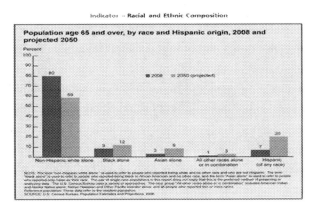

Figure 2. Population age of 65 and over, by race and Hispanic origin 2008 and projected 2050
Source: U.S. Census Bureau, Population Estimates and Projections, 2008

As a percentage, older African–Americans and other racial/ethnic minorities are expected to grow over the same period while older non–Hispanic whites are expected to decline (4). Moreover, life expectancy will continue to climb. In fact, minorities who live to age 85 years have a greater remaining life expectancy than their non–Hispanic white counterparts (the minority aging paradox). And as a subgroup, older African–American females have a similar or greater life expectancy than non–Hispanic white males (5).

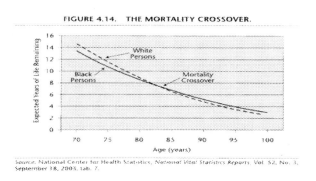

Figure 3. The Mortality Cross Over
Source: National Center for Health Statistics, National Vital Statistics Reports, Vol. 52, No.3, Sept. 18, 2003, tab.7

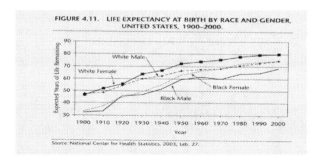

FIGURE 4.11. LIFE EXPECTANCY AT BIRTH BY RACE AND GENDER, UNITED STATES, 1900-2000.

Source: National Center for Health Statistics, 2003, tab. 27.

Socioeconomic burdens of older African-Americans

There have been many explanations for the differences seen in key health indicators for older African-Americans. Most represent continuation in health differences in earlier ages or the accumulation of untoward exposure over an individual's lifetime and beyond.

What are the causes of these disparities? The factors that are associated with health disparities in older adults mirror many of the factors that are associated with health disparities generally. These disparities relate to:

1. Individual Factors
    * Age
    * Genetics
    * Health behaviors
    * Chronic illness
2. Community Factors
    * Education
    * Health care access
    * Community norms
    * Neighborhoods
3. System Factors
    * Health care
    * Local public health
    * Social services
    * Social, economic and health system

These factors are often persistent into late life and contribute to disparities in older populations. The factors that contribute to a difference in the general populations are similar or magnified in older adult populations.

For example, education shows differences across older populations. Both African-Americans and Hispanics show lower high school graduation rates than their older counterparts (7).

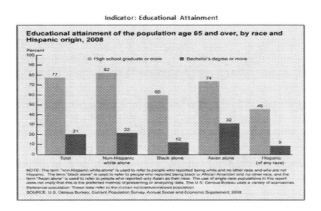

Also, older adults show disparities related to their living arrangements, with African-American men and women being more likely to live alone than other groups (8).

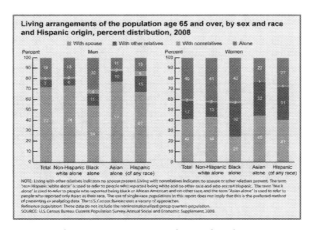

U.S. Census Bureau, Current Population Survey, Annual Social and Economic Supplement, 2008

An alternative explanation for health disparities have been reflected in the area of equal access to health care services. As with younger populations, older African-American show differences in the quality of health care services received (9). These differences led to disparities despite the elimination of significant barrier to access

– health insurance. Many African-Americans once they become 65 years old enroll in Medicare. Thus, they become insured and the barrier of insurance is eliminated. Despite having insurance coverage, older African-Americans show higher rates of amputations for diabetic complications, lower rates of coronary artery bypass grafting and lower rates of kidney transplantation (11). As the model depicted below suggests, perhaps these disparities in older African-American represent systemic issues, prejudice, or racial stereotyping.

Figure 1: Differences, Disparities, and Discrimination: Populations with Equal Access to Health Care

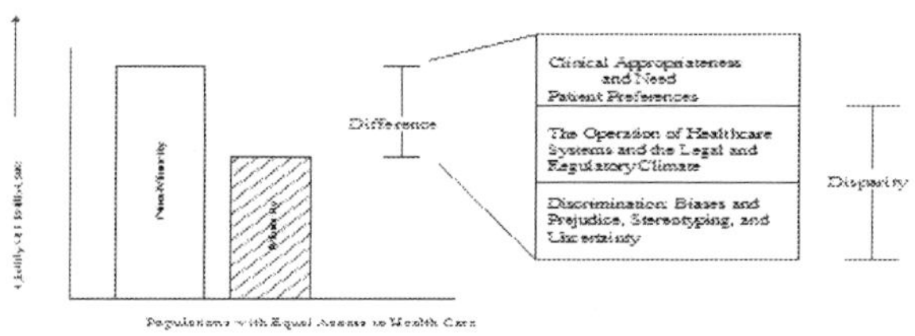

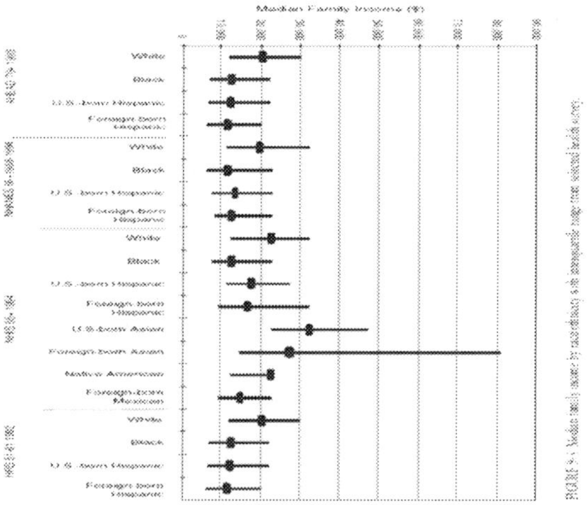

Other causes – Health literacy

Health literacy is an important contributor to health disparities in older adults. In fact, up to 20 percent of Spanish-speaking Latinos do not seek medical advice due to language barriers (14). Asians and Hispanics often report difficulties understanding written information from doctor's offices and instructions on prescription bottles. Up to 40 percent of African-Americans have problems reading (15). Also, over two-thirds of elders 60-plus have low to marginal reading skills. Adults with poor literacy are likely to have three times as many prescriptions filled as adults with higher literacy.

Specific Health Disparities in Older African-Americans

Older U.S. minorities have shorter overall life expectancy (74.3 years for non-Hispanic white males versus 67.2 years for African-American males) and higher rates of cardiovascular disease, cancer, diabetes mellitus and glaucoma (16). As mentioned above, some key contributing factors include reduced access to health care, occupation exposure and socioeconomic factors.

Cardiovascular disease

With regard to cardiovascular disease, older African-Americans have 1.5 times the number of heart disease deaths as their non-Hispanic white counterparts. Black mortality rates are especially elevated for heart disease and cerebrovascular disease and exceed those for whites at any age beyond 44 years (17). For example, African-Americans have 1.3 times the number of nonfatal cerebrovascular accidents and 1.8 times the number of fatal cerebrovascular accidents as their non-Hispanic white counterparts. In addition, African-Americans have five times the rate of end-stage renal disease as their non-Hispanic white counterparts and a lower rate of kidney transplantation (18).

Disability

The rate of chronic disability among black and Native American men at ages 30–34 years is not reached until decades later for whites and Asians (18). Blacks live many fewer years and live many more years with a chronic disability than longest-lived group, Asians. Native Americans live longer, but live an extended period of their lives with disability.

Osteoporosis

The rate of osteoporosis is greatest in non-Hispanic white (and Asian-American) women at approximately 33 percent compared to the lowest rate in African-American women at approximately 25 percent (20). The U.S. Preventive Services Task Force recommends dual X-ray absorptiometry screening in postmenopausal women after 65.

Hip fracture rates are 2-3.2 times higher in non-Hispanic white women versus African-American women.

Glaucoma

Glaucoma is a leading cause of visual impairment in older adults. Older African-Americans have 4-6 times higher rate of glaucoma than non-Hispanic whites (21). The USPSTF recommends screening for glaucoma using measurement of intraocular pressures begin at age 40 years in African-Americans. Another leading cause of blindness, macular degeneration is higher in non-Hispanics whites.

Disparities in prevention

In additional to disease, older adults also have disparities in the utilization of preventive services. For both influenza and pneumococcal vaccination, African-Americans and Hispanics have lower vaccination rates compared to non-Hispanic whites (13).

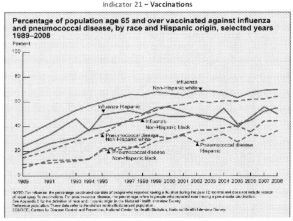

Other screening tests and interventions show disparities

Younger African-American women have had improvement in their mammogram utilization but older African-American women lag behind their non-Hispanic white counterparts (20). Moreover, African-American women are less likely to follow-up on abnormal mammography results than their non-Hispanic white counterparts (11).

Black and White Differences in Specialty Procedure Utilization Among
Medicare Beneficiaries Age 65 and Older, 1993

	Black	White	Black-to-White Ratio
Angioplasty (procedures per 1,000 beneficiaries per year)	2.5	5.4	0.46
Coronary Artery Bypass Graft Surgery (procedures per 1,000 beneficiaries per year)	1.9	4.8	0.40
Mammography (procedures per 100 women per year)	17.1	26.0	0.66
Hip Fracture Repair (procedures per 100 women per year)	2.9	7.0	0.42
Amputation of All or Part of Limb (procedures per 1,000 beneficiaries per year)	6.7	1.9	3.64
Bilateral Orchiectomy (procedures per 1,000 beneficiaries per year)	2.0	0.8	2.45

Source: Gornick et al. 1996

Other screening tests (Dementia, Depression)

In addition, many of the screening tests used to assess older adults showed difference and there utilization should be adjusted to address these differences. In particular, screening for cognitive dysfunction and dementia showed differences based on race. [22] The Mini Mental State Exam (MMSE) shows:

- lower threshold for cognitive impairment in African–American and Hispanics
- cutoff of less 18/30 versus standard 23/30 cutoff
- sensitivity 82 percent, specificity 99 percent

The Short Portable Mental Status Questionnaire has been validated in African–Americans and Hispanic Americans and avoids some of the variability based on race found in the MMSE (23). Other cognitive assessments (i.e. Mini-Cog, Clock Drawing Task) have less racial/ethnic variation and can be reliably used in older African–Americans.

Measures of depression in older adults also show variability according to race/ethnicity. One of the most commonly used instruments, the Geriatric Depression Scale, shows racial/ethnic variation (24). The GDS is less sensitive in African–Americans (75 percent versus 94 percent) and Hispanics than non–Hispanic whites. The Center for Epidemiologic Studies Depression scale (CES-D) has better reliability (0.84–0.92) in older African–Americans and has a Spanish language translation available (24).

How the ACA addresses some the causes on health disparities

The Patient Protection and Affordable Care Act (ACA) (25) has many provisions designed to protect and enhance health care for older adults. Under ACA, Medicare is key vehicle for quality and cost initiatives, i.e. accountability:

- **Goal: Transform Medicare from a passive payer to an active purchaser of higher quality, more efficient health care through:**
  - Value-based purchasing (26)
  - Payment reductions for unnecessary hospital readmissions and hospital-acquired conditions
  - Pilots and Demos

Value-based purchasing arrangements have the potential to provide transparency and monitoring of many of the health outcomes mentioned above. As providers of health services begin to evaluate how well they are providing services to an entire population, variability becomes a more apparent threat to good outcomes. Hopefully, the drive to provide the best outcomes will close the gaps between older adult subpopulations and reduce disparities.

Unnecessary hospitalization also has the potential to drive a reduction in disparities. Avoiding hospitalization in older adults will necessitate an improvement in screening and preventive services as well as better ambulatory management of chronic conditions. Accountable Care Organizations and other providers will need to manage risk and reducing variability is the essential component.

However, monitoring by local, state, or federal government will need to be comprehensive and consistent to avoiding the shifting of high cost populations by health providers or the withholding appropriate treatment due to cost considerations.

What does (should) the ideal future look like

While the ACA and fiscal reform sets the stage from the broad U.S. population to ask, "What is the right kind of health care payment system that provides the best outcomes for older adults?" Of particular interest is the question, "What system ensures the improvement of health and function for older adults while eliminating health disparities in this population?" These questions can be answered by considering what the best care is across the lifespan.

Arguably the greatest improvement in health has resulted in broad public programs (i.e. sanitation, infection control, immunization). And there success perhaps stems from their application to the entire population without regard to race/ethnicity or socioeconomic status. The greatest opportunity for an ideal future and the elimination of health disparities in older adults is a health system change that promoted earlier prevention, appropriate screening and early detection, and easy access to care when needed.

Conclusion

This chapter presents an understanding of the health disparities issues facing older adult populations while discussing the impact that health reform can have on mitigating these disparities. Understanding the factors that impact health disparities in older adults provides the opportunity to eliminate disparities in the current changing health care environment.

References

Compiled by Ekwo Anthony MD, MPH
1. NIH Strategic Research Plan and Budget to Reduce and Ultimately Eliminate Health Disparities, Vol. 1, Fiscal Years 2002–2006.
2. Institute of Medicine. Unequal Treatment: Confronting Racial and Ethnic Disparities in Health Care. Washington, DC: National Academy Press; 2002.
3. Minority Health and Health Disparities Research and Education Act of 2000 (47, page 2498).
4. U.S. Dept. of Commerce, U.S. Census Bureau. (2008) Population projections, 2008. Washington, D.C: Author.
5. National Center for Health Statistics, National Vital Statistics Reports, Vol. 52, No.3, September 18, 2003, tab.7
6. National Center for Health Statistics, National Vital Statistics Reports, Vol. 52, No.3, September 28, 2003, tab.27
7. U.S. Dept. of Commerce, U.S. Census Bureau. (2008) Current Population Survey, Annual Social and Economic Supplement, 2008. Washington, D.C: Author.
8. U.S. Department of Health and Human Services, Office of Minority Health (2011). Disparities Reduction Efforts. Washington, D.C. 20013-7337
9. Institute of Medicine (2002). Guidance for the National Healthcare Disparities Report, p.99
10. Office of Disease Prevention and Health Promotion. 2002. *Healthy People 2010.* US Department of Health and Human Services 2001.
11. Gornick M.E., Eggers P.W., Reilly T.W., et al. Effects of race and income on mortality and use of services among Medicare beneficiaries. N Engl J Med 1996; 335:791-799.
12. Jones J., (1990). Black-white disparities in health care. JAMA 1990; 263:2344–6.
13. Center for Disease Control and Prevention (2008). Percentage of Population age 65 and Over Vaccinated against Influenza and Pneumococcal disease by race and Hispanic origin. Aging Trends Website Available at www.cdc.gov/nchs/agingact.htm.

14. US Dept Health and Human Services (2003), National Healthcare Disparities Report. Retrieved on 4/24/13 from http://www.cfah.org/factsoflife/vol8no3.cfm

15. Institute of Medicine. (2009). *Toward health equity and patient-centeredness: Integrating health literacy, disparities reduction, and quality improvement: Workshop summary.* Washington, DC: National Academies Press.

16. US Census Bureau, (2005). Current Population Report, Special Studies. Annual Social and Economic Supplement, p.209

17. Keppel, K., Pearcy, J., & Wagener, D. (2002). Trends in racial and ethnic-specific rates for health status indicators: United States, 1990-98. *Health People 2000.* Statistical Notes: Number 23; Centers for Disease Control.

18. Mouton, C. (1997). Special health considerations in African-American elders. *American Family Physician,* 55, 1243-1253

19. Wong, M., et.al. (2002). Contribution of major diseases to disparities in mortality. *New England Journal of Medicine,* 347:1585-1592.

20. Weisman, C. (1998). *Women's Health Care.* Baltimore, MD: John Hopkins University Press.

21. Richardson, J. (1996). *Aging and Health: Black American Elders,* (2nd ed.) SGEC Working Paper # 4. Stanford, CA: Stanford GEC.

22. Clark PC, Kutner NG, Goldstein FC, et al., (2005). Impediments to timely diagnosis of Alzheimer's disease in African Americans. *J Am Geriatr Soc.* 2005 Nov;53 (11):2012-7.

23. Mouton, C. & Esparza, Y.B. (2001). Ethnicity and Geriatric Assessment. In J. Gallo, T. Fulmer, G. J. Paveza, & W. Reichel (Eds.) *Handbook of Geriatric Assessment* (pp. 1–28). Gaithersburg, MD: Aspen Publishers

24. Mouton, C.P., Johnson, M.S., & Cole, D.R. (1995). Ethical considerations with African-American elders. *Clinics in Geriatric Medicine,* 11, 113–129.

25. U.S. House of Representatives, (2010). Compilation of Patient Protection and *Affordable Care Act,* 111th Congress, 2d Session.

26. Center for Medicare and Medicaid Services, (2012). **Roadmap for Implementing Value Driven Healthcare in the Traditional Medicare Fee-for-Service Program. Retrieved April 25, 2013 from http://www.cms.gov/Medicare/Quality-Initiatives-Patient-Assessment-Instruments/QualityInitiativesGenInfo/downloads/vbproadmap_oea_1-16_508.pdf**

CHAPTER 10
NMA and the Value of Global Outreach

Coauthor: Hilary Akpudo, MD

Over the years, the National Medical Association has taken a more global view of health care issues, concerns and challenges. Natural disasters, such as earthquakes, hurricanes and tsunamis can overwhelm a strong health care system in an established country. For a poor nation, it could mean a disaster that could pummel that nation for generations to come.

In 2012, the National Medical Association established a relationship with the country of Liberia. The West African country has made strides after years of civil wars and coups. Liberia and African-Americans, of course, have some natural roots. The country was colonized by former U.S. slaves returning to Africa beginning in 1820, and it was one of two sub-Saharan African countries not colonized by Europe. President Ellen Johnson Sirleaf, the winner of the 2011 Nobel Peace Prize in particular saw the connection between Liberia's hopes and the NMA's global mission. Some 85 percent of Liberians continue to live below the international poverty line.

"The services you provided to our people during your stay in Liberia have given us belief that we can always work together to do more for the people, and this is why we promise you total commitment in providing an enabling environment in your humanitarian work," she said during our NMA visit in November of 2012.

Doctors and nurses from NMA, which included health care workers from across the United States, visited the country for a week, providing medical assistance to needy Liberians for free. They worked in collaboration with the Liberia Medical and Dental Association (LMDA).

In early 2013, the NMA made a second trip to Liberia, bringing 37 physicians to the country, where they performed surgeries, taught students and gave medical guidance to the country's health care leaders.

The need for physicians and physician training in Liberia come at a critical time. Index Mundi.com, which compiles statistical data on various countries, ranks Liberia 187 out of 188 countries in the number of doctors per its population. Liberia has 0.01 doctors per 1,000 residents. The United States, for example, has 2.67 physicians per 1,000 residents. Cuba has 6.40 physicians per 1,000 residents. A September, 2012 story by the Washington Post Writers Group noted that 12 of 15 counties in Liberia have no doctor at all to serve its residents (5).

It's against this backdrop that the National Medical Association has recently signed a letter of memorandum with the Liberian government to provide medical training to doctors and nurses. NMA is also playing a role in generating support to get a medical school started in the country and encouraging native Liberian medical students to return to their homeland.

NMA members have been working with former U.S. Health and Human Services secretary Dr. Louis Sullivan and the World Bank to bring additional medical training in Liberia. As of April of 2013, the World Bank has committed $20 million for postgraduate medical school training there. NMA has approached the World Bank and Eric Goosby, the U.S. Global AIDS coordinator who directs the President's Emergency Plan for AIDS Relief (PEPFAR), with a request for additional funds.

Cuba and Universal Health Care

NMA members visited Cuba from Feb. 10-17, 2013 for a government-approved professional exchange with Cuban physicians. It was an eye-opening experience. The trip was organized by former NMA president Dr. Rodney Hood (NMA president 2000). Dr. Hood, a distinguished physician in San Diego, Calif., has led these professional exchanges for numerous years. In 2011, he was honored with the Pride in the Profession Award from the American Medical Association Foundation for his work with the underserved population in the United States.

He started leading these exchanges at the request of the Congressional Black Caucus. In the past, his delegations have included former U.S. Surgeon Generals Dr. Joycelyn Elders and Dr. Julius B. Richmond. February's delegation included myself, along with former NMA presidents Dr. Winston Price, of New York (NMA president 2004), and Dr. Richard Butcher, of California (NMA president 1992).

There is no other place in the world that has a higher density of physicians per 1,000 residents than Cuba (6.40 per 1,000 residents) (6). Our delegation reviewed the notable differences between the U.S. and Cuba health care system and what can be learned and shared with the Cuban physicians and medical professionals we visited.

Cuba has universal health care coverage. What Cuba does well that we can carry to the U.S. is coordinated and integrated care. With coordinated and integrated care, doctors and other health care professionals work together to treat the patient on all levels. This created a comprehensive system of "checks and balances" for the patient and his or her health care needs.

The challenge for Cuba is that it is a relatively poor country. While the country's medical community makes due with what it has, it doesn't have the latest medical equipment to serve its citizens in the highest quality possible. In my opinion, continued exchanges with Cuban physicians will play a great role in improving medical services in both countries.

Outreach in Botswana

Meharry Medical College, the largest private historically black institution dedicated to health care education in the country, has established a relation with the country of Botswana. Meharry President Wayne J. Riley, MD, MBA was the keynote speaker at the convocation for the first class of medical students at the University of Botswana Medical School. Those students are expected to complete their studies in 2014.

"This is a significant milestone in the long journey toward attaining a doctor of medicine," Dr. Riley said at the convocation. "Having the opportunity to represent Meharry Medical College during this momentous occasion is both an honor and a privilege. Our missions are aligned as both UB and Meharry strive to meet the health care needs of the underserved and underrepresented."

Crisis in Haiti

These global efforts are often put to the test in some of the world's greatest crises. Doctors from the National Medical Association have seen such a situation in the aftermath of the January 2010 earthquake in Haiti. A 7.0 magnitude earthquake rocked that country on Jan. 10, causing widespread damage throughout the country, including the crowded national capital of Port-Au-Prince. Haiti was slowly recovering from past hurricanes and tropical storms, making the destruction of the earthquake near catastrophic.

In an article for the Journal for the Poor and Underserved, I described the desperate conditions in Haiti weeks after the earthquake and how basic health care efforts and organization made a tangible difference for the people the NMA provided help for.

Haiti is the poorest country in the Western Hemisphere, with limited infrastructure and makeshift dwellings. Death figures are estimated at 250,000. In 2012, more than 500,000 continued to live in temporary shelters with no sign of when permanent residences will be constructed for them. It was against that backdrop that many relief workers – including doctors from many organizations including the National Medical Association – provided care and probably most importantly, hope.

On Jan. 28, 2010, doctors went on a disaster relief mission to Haiti under the joint auspices of Arise and Walk Ministries Foundation (2), and Bethel Gospel Assembly. The NMA led similar relief efforts after Hurricane Katrina hit New Orleans and the Gulf Coast in August 2005. The Arise and Walk Ministries Foundation is a disaster relief organization led by Mark J. Wade, MD, a pediatrician based in Newark, N.J. Dr. Wade is the founder and CEO of Wade Healthcare Systems, Inc. (WHS), a physician-owned and operated health care management and consultation company. At the time, he was a member of the NMA Board of Directors.

Arise and Walk Ministries Foundation is a Christian-based ministry whose mission is to equip and empower the local church with the health care personnel, expertise and resources necessary to provide health care excellence as an integral part of their missionary outreach to the nations of the world. Bethel Gospel Assembly, under the leadership of Bishop Carlton Theophilus Brown, is a Christian church based in Harlem. Bethel Gospel Assembly Ministries includes six churches in Transkei, South Africa. Bishop Brown served in mission assignments.

The NMA, Arise and Walk Ministries Foundation, and Bethel Gospel Assembly worked with other professional and philanthropic organizations for ongoing support for Haiti. The goal is to nurture long-standing relationships and build resources that will help the Haitian people rebuild their lives.

I led the NMA team to Santo Domingo, Dominican Republic on Thursday, Jan. 28, 2010 amidst concern about security in Haiti. There were reports that all of the country's prisoners had to be released following the earthquake. Another group ahead of us had reportedly been intercepted by an unidentified armed militia. Haitian police, a group of four armed policemen wielding semiautomatic rifles, provided escort for the NMA team. The United Nations Security forces walked the streets, providing strong command presence. Their presence certainly helped bring a sense of stability to the pervasive feeling of vulnerability.

My team brought needed supplies to the helpless and stranded people of Haiti. The supplies included food, bottled water, wheel chairs, medical and surgical supplies, and volunteer medical, surgical, and psychiatric resources experts. The Grace Catholic Church/Orphanage, which housed 200 girls, had no running water, no plumbing, and only a three-day supply of food.

There were reportedly 18,000 people living inside the preliminary barrier gate of the church. People bathed in the open, kids were naked and the makeshift tents in which they lived were barely erect. The feelings of vulnerability and hopelessness were palpable. The need for food, shelter, health care, and psychological support among these displaced and devastated people was brutally obvious.

These people were badly in need of psychiatrists who could help them cope with their psychological torment, anxiety and depression. They asked, "How can things possibly get better?" It was a difficult, but appropriate, question. We provided opportunities for groups to talk, to address their respective concerns, in a kind of on-the-ground psychotherapy. It was rudimentary at best, but beneficial. Participants expressed a motivation to live through the difficulty until things improve.

Post-Traumatic Stress Disorder (PTSD) is often diagnosed in people who have been through the experience of war. Psychiatrically, in Haiti, a large number of individuals most likely met the diagnostic criteria for PTSD pre-earthquake. The earthquake itself added a clearly catastrophic stressor to create a new paradigm in disaster relief and recovery. There was a need to better understand the full impact of this type of psychological assault on an individual's psychological defense mechanisms.

It stands to reason that any individual who has been so affected has fewer emotional reserves available to be able to address the primary day-to-day struggles to which he or she are exposed. Depressive and anxiety disorders can be very debilitating, especially in individuals with poor pre-morbid functioning (4). This is the case in Haiti. Social and economic deprivations, with all its ugly ramifications, had pervaded these people before the devastating earthquake added insult to injury.

Dr. Riley has been, and continues to be, a powerful ally in this most important endeavor.

The support of Dr. Billy Ray Ballard, interim dean, School of Medicine, and Interim Vice President, of Health Affairs, Meharry Medical College, made it possible to work around administrative hurdles that might have derailed the Haiti project. Ms. Lori B. Donnell, executive director, Meharry Medical Group Administration used her extensive network to provide much of the medical supplies taken by our team on the Haiti trip.

The donations from Meharry — including food, bottled water, cleaning solutions (e.g., Betadine and alcohol), bandages, personal hygiene items (feminine), antibiotics, surgical and orthopedic supplies, and even a tent—were very well received.

While the situation in Haiti has improved, many Haitians continue to survive in the same conditions they lived in immediately after the earthquake. The NMA made a difference but it drove home the point of continued global outreach. Health care services in many respects are just as, and even more, important than brick-and-mortar projects. Proper health care gives people not only the better mental capacity and wellness to improve the conditions around them, but it also gives them and their families hope.

References

1. U.S. Geological Survey. Magnitude 7.0—Haiti region. Reston, VA: USGS National Center, 2010. Available at: http://earthquake.usgs.gov/eqcenter/eqinthenews/2010/ us2010rja6/.

2. Arise and Walk Ministries Foundation. Arise and walk ministries foundation mission and vision. Paramus, NJ, 2009. Available at: http://www.awmfoundation.org/about_us/ mission vision. shtml.

3. Bethel Gospel Assembly. About Bethel Gospel Assembly. New York, NY: Bethel Gospel Assembly, 2010. Available at: http://www.bethelga.org/mission.aspx.

4. DepressionIsReal.org. Separating fact from fiction: offering help and hope. 2009. Available at: http://ww-w.depressionisreal.org/podcast/bio_bailey.php.

5. Michael Gerson, Washington Post Writers Group, Miami Herald, "Fighting childhood deaths, Liberia chooses life." http://www.miamiherald.com/2012/06/24/2863799/fighting-childhood-deaths-liberia.html.

6. Index Mundi.com. Demographics: Country Comparison. Physician Density. http://www.indexmundi.com/g/r.aspx?v=2226

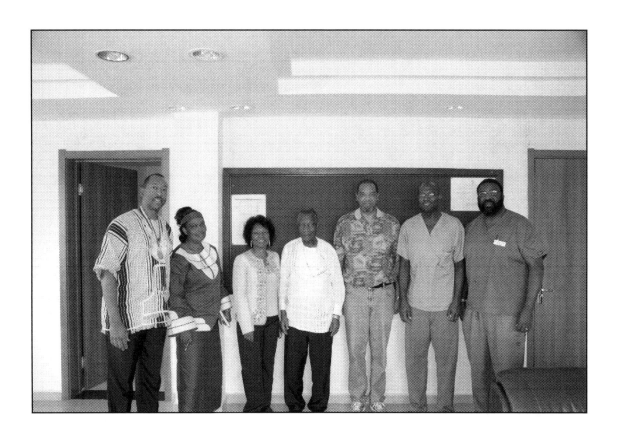

From left to right: Dr. Bailey with Deputy Minister of Health for Liberia, Dr. Anita Jackson, Minister of Health- Dr. Walter T. Gwenigale, Dr. Greg Antoine, Dr. Qualls Stevens and Dr. Frank Glover.

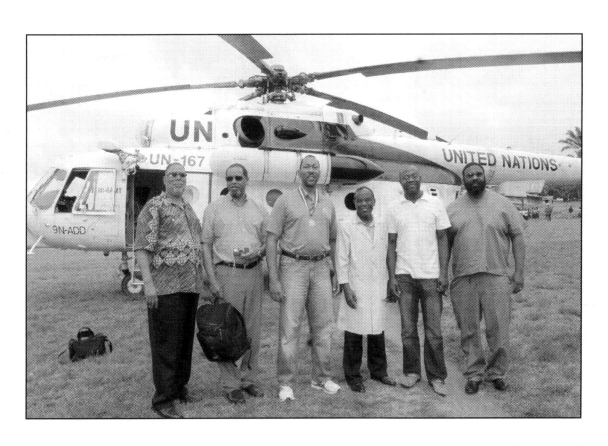

Dr. Bailey with a team of doctors prepare to fly to Jackson F. Doe Memorial Regional Referral Hospital in Tappita, Nimba County, Liberia.

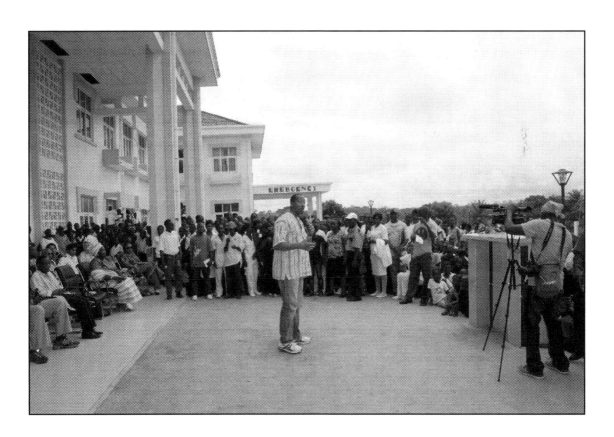

Dr. Bailey gives a speech in front of a crowd of about a thousand people in front of the Jackson F. Doe Memorial Regional Referral Hospital. The $10 million, 206-bed facility was built in 2011 to honor the late educator and politician. Photo by Frank Glover, MD.

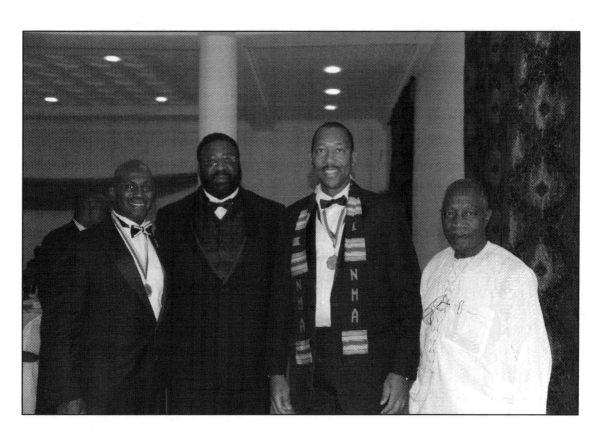

From left to right, Dr. Leonard Weather, Dr. Frank Glover, Dr. Bailey and Dr. Walter T. Gwenigale (Minister of Health and Social Welfare for Liberia).

CHAPTER 11
Summation

Critical issues about the health care system in the United States have been around since the founding of the country more than 230 years ago. From the doctor with his little black bag making house calls, to some of the world's greatest advances curing diseases once considered incurable, the profession has taken giant leaps.

Yet, issues of health care disparities, stigma and access to services continue to prevent health care in this country from reaching its true potential for all Americans. That is one of the reasons these issues have been a major theme of the National Medical Association.

Below is a summation of these issues the NMA hopes will continue to receive a full debate as the country continues to wrestle with what is the best way to distribute health care to its citizens.

Elimination of Health Care Disparities

The Connecticut Health Disparities Project describes health care disparities as the avoidable differences in disease burden and health outcomes among specific population groups that result from cumulative social disadvantages. These differences are based on race, ethnicity, age, gender, socioeconomic position, immigration status, sexual orientation, language, disability, disease status, homelessness and geographical area of residence. These disparities occur either due to the way the society is structured or as a result of biased treatment by the health care system. The result is that there is the "continual accumulation of unfavorable health events" impacting the disadvantaged populations. These unfavorable health events not only lead to poor health outcomes, they also manifest themselves in different areas of life, including:

- Familial and social relationships
- Housing
- Neighborhood
- Environmental
- Occupational conditions
- Societal expressions of discrimination
- Opportunity, and
- Health care access (1).

These biases may be conscious or unconscious. But disparities are not only harmful to disadvantaged populations. They affect the entire population negatively not only morally, but from an economic standpoint as well. In a report by the Joint Center for Political and Economic Studies, researchers from Johns Hopkins University and the University of Maryland-Baltimore reported the United States lost about $229 billion between 2003 and 2006 because disparities in treatment and care that could have been prevented (3).

"The statistics are just stunning and shocking," said Kathleen Sebelius, the Secretary of Health and Human Services, during the announcement of the findings. "There is no question that reducing the health disparities can save incredible amounts of money. But more importantly, it saves lives and it makes us a healthier and more prosperous nation (4)."

This makes the elimination of health care disparities even more urgent because not only do disparities make us unhealthy as a nation, but they also make us poorer economically. It is for this reason that eliminating health care disparities should be considered a top priority.

Removing the Sigma of Mental Illness

Stigma results from individual and societal misunderstanding of the nature and presentation of mental illness. People with mental illness often have to struggle to deal with symptoms of mental illness as well as the societal stigma toward them. Thus, mental illness affects individuals in overcoming difficulties in coping with symptoms of the disease and the disadvantages caused by societal reactions to those individuals (5). Several studies revealed that stigma generally arose from lack of awareness, lack of perception, and the nature and complications of mental illness (6).

It is experienced universally, that isolates people with mental illness and delays in the treatment of individuals. That often results in a massive social and economic burden (7). Many individuals who might receive mental health services do not obtain them fully or adhere to treatment regimens once the individual has received treatment. Treatment adherence plays a vital role in psychiatric rehabilitation (8).

Stigma related to schizophrenia is particularly high (9). Behavioral symptoms associated with schizophrenia play the main role in stigmatization. Some 69 percent of patients felt that stigma arose from attitudes in the general community, 46 percent from co-workers and 42 percent from family members (10).

Several advocacy groups have developed strategies to target various components of stigma. These strategies are grouped into the three processes: protest, education and contact (11).

Stigma is presented as a type of moral injustice through protest and people are discouraged from acting in these socially inappropriate ways. Organized protest can be useful to convince the media to stop stigmatized representations (12). Stigma Busters is a protest group which is a part of the National Alliance on Mental Illness (NAMI). It has more than 15,000 national and international advocates who work together on the Internet (13). The members respond to stigmatized portrayals in various media that influence Americans by disapproval and encouragement to boycott (13). In 2000, it took a prominent role to persuade the ABC network to cancel the program "Wonderland" which portrayed persons with mental illness as dangerous and unpredictable (12).

The Center for Mental Health Services developed the group called Elimination of Barrier Initiative (EBI), which had as its mandate in educating the public to challenge the stigma of mental illness. The goal of this three-year project was to combat discrimination, reduce barriers to treatment, and build public support for recovery. Evaluations of this project showed encouraging results. The dissemination of EBI's public service announcement, "Mental Health: It's Part of Our Lives" was impressive. A total of 7,306 commitments for broadcasts and cable use of public service announcements (representing a possible viewing audience of 150 million) were received. Print advertisements of EBI had been circulated by 120 newspapers and 11 magazines represented circulation of more than four million (14).

The third and most effective strategy to combat stigma is contact. People with mental illness have access to the In Our Own Voice program to challenge public stigma. In this approach, face-to-face and interpersonal contact between a person with mental illness and the general public takes place (15). It is a 90-minute standardized contact program in which persons with mental illness interact with an audience on topics involving mental illness. It is also a program of NAMI (16).

The three above approaches possess several merits that endorse the fight against mental illness stigma. There are some preliminary research projects that offer initial support to the feasibility and usefulness of these programs. However, more data and research are needed to fully establish these approaches as evidence-based practices. Mental health care professionals, primary health care professionals, patients and their families are required to get involved actively to eliminate stigma against those who suffer from mental illness. The more these stakeholders work together, the more efficient they will be.

Enabling Access to Health Care

Access to health care in America has always been a controversial issue. Some believe health care should be available to all, irrespective of race, economic or social factors. Others comment on the cost restraints of such open access. Access to appropriate health care resources is necessary to preserve and improve the health care of people in general (17). In the opinion of the National Medical Association, access to quality health care must be a basic human right.

Previous literature has shown deterioration in access to medical care for certain groups of people. That is particularly the case for minorities, the uninsured and the indigent. According to one health care survey, for these groups "the overall health care use and per person physician visits declined by 22 percent (18)." The problem is a large portion of Americans do not have a primary care physician. It has been estimated that about four out of five persons who are currently uninsured actually work.

Health care involves services that include medical care, dental care, eye care, prescription medicine and mental health. Factors related to health care access include family income, race/ethnicity, health insurance and place of residence. Health insurance continues to be an important factor influencing access to medical care. In one key study, the number of physician visits was remarkably low for the uninsured as compared to the insured (22).

A substantial number of Americans have underused medical and dental services. This could be due to social and cultural values or lack of understanding for appropriate use of care. Public awareness programs to improve education should therefore be supplemented.

Public attention has brought a greater focus on racial and ethnic disparities in regards to health care access. African-Americans and Hispanics were found to have the highest percentage of uninsured. That drastically limits these two groups' access to quality health care (19).

Immigrants, a growing part of American society, face even greater difficulties in this regard (20). They have disproportionally lower incomes, which increase their risk of being uninsured. That concern subsequently furthers limits their access to even the most basic form of health care. There exists a need to have better access to health care and to reduce barriers to care. The language barrier was found to be one of the most common. The lack of English proficiency for immigrants has led to misdiagnosis and under treatment (21). Interpreters and translation services should therefore be utilized to minimize the chance of errors.

Residents of rural communities and some in the inner cities may have compromised access to health care because of geographical location. It is a national goal to close the rural/urban gap for health care service. The Patient Protection and Affordable Care Act has the potential to address all of these concerns. More than 30 million uninsured Americans should now have access to a system of quality basic health care.

Members of the National Medical Association have come to realize that the more people are involved in the health care system, the better the medical profession will be and the stronger the nation will be. By standing united for this care, the NMA looks to a better future not only for ethnic minorities and the poor, but for all Americans.

References

1. Stratton A, Hynes M, Nepaul A. The Connecticut Healthcare Disparities Project: Connecticut Department of Public Health, Hartford, Conn., Summer 2007.
2. Sabin J, Nosek BA, Greenwald A., Rivara FP. Journal of Healthcare for the Poor and Underserved: 2009, August 20(3); 893-913.
3. LaVeist TA, Gaskin DJ, Richard P. The Economic Burden of Health Inequities in the United States. Joint Center for Political and Economic Studies: September 2009.
4. The Baltimore Sun. Friday, September 19, 2009.
5. Rusch H, Angermeyer MC, Corrigan PW. Mental illness stigma: Concepts, consequences, and initiatives to reduce stigma. European Psychiatry. 2005, 20: 529-539.
6. Ardoleda-Flore z J: What causes stigma? World Psychiatry. 2002, 1: 25-6.
7. Shrivastava A, Johnston M, Bureau Y: Stigma of Mental Illness-1: Clinical reflections. Mens Sana Monographs. 2012, 10(1): 70-85.
8. Tsang HW, Fung KM, Corrigan PW. Psychosocial treatment compliance scale for people with psychotic disorders. Aust NZ J Psychiatry. 2006, 40:561-9.

9. Thara R. Srinivasan TN. How stigmatizing is schizophrenia in India? Int J Soc Psychiatry. 2000, 46: 135-41.

10. Shrivastava A, Johnson ME, Thakar M, Shrivastava S, Sarkhel G, Sunita I et al: Orgin and impact of stigma and discrimination in schizophrenia-patients' perception. Mumbai study. Stigma Research Action. 2001, 1: 67-72.

11. Corrigan PW, Penn DL. Lessons from social psychology on discrediting psychiatric stigma. American Psychologist, 1999, 54: 765-776.

12. Corrigan PW, Gelb B. Three Programs That Use Mass Approaches to Challenge the Stigma of Mental Illness. Psychiatric Services. 2006, 57: 393-398.

13. Corrigan PW, Watson AC. At Issue: Stop: Call mental illness a brain disease. Schizophrenia Bulletin. 2004, 30: 477-479.

14. Troust D. On the Elimination of Barriers Initiative. Personal Contact, 2005.

15. Pettigrew TF, Tropp, LR. Does intergroup contact reduce prejudice: recent meta-analytic findings, in Reducing Prejudice and Discrimination. Edited by Oskamp S. Mahawah. N.J., Erlbaum, 2000.

16. Corrigan PW: On the Stigma of Mental Illness. American Psychological Association, Washington, D.C., 2005.

17. Gulliford M, Figueroa-Munoz J, Morgan M, Hughes D, Gibson B, Beech R, Hudson M. J Health Serv Res Policy, July1, 2002. Vol. 7, No. 3: 186-188.

18. Haffner SM, Fong D, Stern MP, Pugh JA, Hazuda HP, Patterson JK, Van Heuven WAJ, Klein R. Diabetic retinopathy in Mexican-Americans and non-Hispanic whites. Diabetes 37: 878-884, 1988.

19. U.S. Commission on Civil Rights, The Health Care Challenge: Acknowledging Disparities, Confronting Discrimination; Vol. I, The Role of Government and Private Health Care Programs and Intiatives.

20. Kaiser Commission on Medicaid and the Uninsured, Immigrants Health Care: Coverage and access (Washington: Kaiser Family Foundation, Aug. 2000).

21. Flores G, et al. Access Barriers to Health Care for Latino Children. Archives of Pediatric and Adolescent Medicine 152. No. 11 (1998): 1119-1125.

22. Committee on the Cost of Medical Care, Medical Care for the American People (New York: Arno Press, 1972), 8.

Epilogue
A Letter of Greeting

Greetings my colleagues and associates in the health care profession. We are here to make America a healthier nation by making sure that every American enjoys basic, affordable, comprehensive health care, irrespective of race, ethnicity, age, gender, sexual orientation, immigration status, or financial circumstance. I commend your commitment and steadfastness in this struggle. We dedicate ourselves to the cause of providing health care to the poor, the underserved, the neglected and the forgotten in our culture.

During this year as the NMA's 113th president, based on my abiding principle in life that "where there are problems, let's solve them," I decided to focus on three areas that are of great importance to me personally and to us as an association. These are the areas of reforming health care, eliminating disparities and removing stigma. With recent developments, controlling gun violence has become an essential addition to this list. This book represents an important milestone in finding solutions to these very serious problems.

I especially applaud you for being true physicians for refusing to look the other way when you saw your fellow Americans in dire straits. Every day you willingly engage your patients to ensure that we become a healthier and better country, and a healthier and better people. You are making a great difference in people's lives.

The difference a physician can make can be the difference between good health and disease, and even between life and death. I encourage you to remain strong and committed to the course you have chosen, because you are on the right track.

There may be times when what you do may seem unappreciated. You may conduct your work anonymously, but I assure you, you are not anonymous to the ones you help (and their families), or the lives you help change and save. We recognize that you do not do these things for fame or fortune. Your reward is the lives you change, the joy you bring to your patients and their families, and the personal fulfillment you get from providing the care that keeps your fellow Americans healthy.

President Barack Obama stated in his second inaugural, "We remember the lessons of our past, when twilight years were spent in poverty and parents of a child with a disability had nowhere to turn. We do not believe that in this country freedom is reserved for the lucky or happiness for the few. We recognize that no matter how responsibly we live our lives, any one of us at any time may face a job loss or a sudden illness or a home swept away in a terrible storm. The commitments we make to each other through Medicare and Medicaid and Social Security, these things do not sap our initiative. They strengthen us. They do not make us a nation of takers. They free us to take the risks that make this country great."

He was probably thinking of a time in the not too distant past, before we had Social Security, Medicare and Medicaid. Many who had put in a lifetime of work lost all that they had, with no means for their health care. Through no fault of their own, many were left at the mercy of a system that had suddenly turned brutal. President Franklin D. Roosevelt signed Social Security into law in 1935 in a step to remedy that problem. President Lyndon B. Johnson went a step farther when he ushered in Medicare and Medicaid in the 1960s.

We don't do things because of a popularity vote. You do them because they are the right things to do. That is why as an association we were also among the first to strongly support the Patient Protection and Affordable Care Act. We believe basic health care should be a right for every American.

Others should be encouraged you to engage with the same mindset in our fight to eliminate health care disparities. As an African-American psychiatrist, I've experienced the impact of disparities on racial and ethnic minorities as well as those who suffer from mental illness. The Affordable Care Act goes a long way to address the problem of disparities. There is still more ground to cover. The existence of disparities represents evidence that the playing field is not yet level.

Finally, there is the issue of stigma. Stigma plays an important role in preventing people who suffer from all forms of illness from coming forward to receive treatment. As knowledge increases, we are gradually accepting that mental illness is just as disabling as physical illness, and that both are illnesses that need to be addressed. In the past, there were physical illnesses that could not be revealed by sufferers because of the stigma they attracted. I have a personal experience of my own grandmother. She suffered from breast cancer and would not tell anyone. By the time we found out, it was too late to save her life. Such is the nature of stigma. As physicians who also understand the deadly impact of stigma, I trust that you will confront it with the same zeal with which you confront increasing health care access and disparities.

God bless you and the National Medical Association.

Blazing the Trail for African-American Doctors
NMA Presidents – Past to Present

1895-1997—Robert F. Boyd, MD
Nashville, Tenn.

1898-1900—H.T. Noel, MD
Nashville, Tenn.

1901-1902—O.D. Porter, MD
Bowling Green, Ky.

1903—F.A. Stewart, MD
Nashville, Tenn.

1904—Charles V. Roman, MD
Dallas, Texas

1905—John E. Hunter, MD
Lexington, Ky.

1906—R.E. Jones, MD
Richmond, Va.

1907—Nathan F. Mossell, MD
Philadelphia, Pa.

1908—W.H. Wright, MD
Baltimore, Md.

1909—P.A. Johnson, MD
New York, N.Y.

1910—Marcus F. Wheatland, MD
Newport, R.I.

1911—Austin M. Curtis, MD
Washington, D.C.

1912—H.F. Gamble, MD
Charles, W.V.

1913—John A. Kenney, Sr., MD
Tuskegee Institute, Ala.

1914—A.M. Brown, MD
Birmingham, Ala.

1915—F.S. Hargraves, MD
Wilson, N.C.

1916—Ulysses G. Dailey, MD
Chicago, Ill.

1917—D.W. Byrd, MD
Norfolk, Va.

1918—George W. Cabaniss, MD
Washington, D.C.

1919—D.A. Ferguson, DDS
Richmond, Va.

1920—J.W. Jones, MD
Winston-Salem, N.C.

1921—John P. Turner, MD
Philadelphia, Pa.

1922—H.M. Green, MD
Knoxville, Tenn.

1923—J. Edward Perry, MD
Kansas City, Mo.

1924—John O. Plummer, MD
Raleigh, N.C.

1925—Michael Q. Dumas, MD
Washington, D.C.

1926—Walter G. Alexander, MD
Orange, N.J.

1927—Carl G. Roberts, MD
Chicago, Ill.

1928—C.V. Freeman, DDS
Jacksonville, Fla.

1929—T. Spotuas Burwell, MD
Philadelphia, Pa.

1930—L.A. West, MD
Memphis, Tenn.

1931—W.H. Higgins, MD
Providence, R.I.

1932—Peter M. Murray, MD
New York, N.Y.

1933—G. Hamilton Francis, MD
Norfolk, Va.

1934—Midian O. Bousfield, MD
Chicago, Ill.

1935—John H. Hale, MD
Nashville, Tenn.

1936—W. Harry Barnes, MD
Philadelphia, Pa.

1937—Roscoe C. Giles, MD
Chicago, Ill.

1938—Lyndon M. Hill, MD
Atlanta, Ga.

1939—George W. Bowles, MD
York, Pa.

1940—Albert W. Dumas, Sr., MD
Natchez, Miss.

1941—Kenneth W. Clement, MD
Cleveland, Ohio

1942—Arthur N. Vaughn, MD
St. Louis, Mo.

1943—Henry Eugene Lee, MD
Houston, Texas

1944-1945—T. Manuel Smith, MD
Chicago, Ill.

1946—Emory I. Robinson, MD
Los Angeles, Calif.

1947—Walter A. Young, MD
St. Louis, Mo.

1948—J.A.C. Lattimore, MD
Louisville, Ky.

1949—C. Austin Whittier, MD
San Antonio, Texas

1950—C. Herbert Marshall, MD
Washington, D.C.

1951—Henry H. Walker, MD
Nashville, Tenn.

1952—Joseph G. Gathings, MD
Washington, D.C.

1953—Whitter C. Atkinson, MD
Coatesville, Pa.

1954—A. Porter Davis, MD
Kansas City, Mo.

1955—Matthew Walker, MD
Nashville, Tenn.

1956—A.C. Terrence, MD
Opelousas, La.

1957—T.R.M. Howard, MD
Chicago, Ill.

1958—Arthur M. Townsend, Jr., MD
St. Louis, Mo.

1959—R. Stillman Smith, MD
Macon, Ga.

1960—Edward C. Mazique, MD
Washington, D.C.

1961—James T. Aldrich, MD
St. Louis, Mo.

1962—Vaughn C. Mason, MD
New York, N.Y.

1963—John A. Kenney, Jr., MD
Washington, D.C.

1964—W. Montague Cobb, MD
Washington, D.C.

1965—Leonidas H. Berry, MD
Chicago, Ill.

1966—John L.S. Hollomon, Jr., MD
New York, N.Y.

1967—Lionel F. Swan, MD
Detroit, Mich.

1968—James M. Whittico, Jr., MD
St. Louis, Mo.

1969—Julius W. Hill, MD
Los Angeles, Calif.

1970—W.T. Armstrong, MD
Rocky Mount, N.C.

1971—Emerson C. Walden, Sr. MD
Baltimore, Md.

1972—Edmund C. Casey, MD
Cincinnati, Ohio

1973—Emery L. Rann, MD
Charlotte, N.C.

1974—Vernal G. Cave, MD
Brooklyn, N.Y.

1975—Jasper F. Williams, MD
Chicago, Ill.

1976—Arthur H. Coleman, MD
San Francisco, Calif.

1977—Charles C. Bookert, MD
Clairton, Pa.

1978—Jesse B. Barber, Jr., MD
Washington, D.C.

1979—Robert Dawson, MD
Durham, N.C.

1980—Vertis R. Thompson, MD
Oakland, Calif.

1981—Frank S. Royal, Sr., MD
Richmond, Va.

1982—Robert L.M. Hilliard, MD
San Antonio, Texas

1983—Lucius C. Earles, III, MD
Chicago, Ill.

1984—Phillip M. Smith, MD
Los Angeles, Calif.

1985—Edith Irby Jones, MD, MACP
Houston, Texas

1986—John O. Brown, MD
Miami, Fla.

1987—John E. Joyner, MD
Indianapolis, Ind.

1988—Frank E. Staggers. Sr., MD
Oakland, Calif.

1989—Vivian W. Pinn, MD
Washington, D.C.

1990—Charles Johnson, MD
Durham, N.C.

1991—Alma Rose George, MD
Detroit, Mich.

1992—Richard O. Butcher, MD
El Cajon, Calif.

1993—Leonard E. Lawrence, MD
San Antonio, Texas

1994—Tracy M. Walton, Jr., MD
Washington, D.C.

1995—Yvonnecris Smith Veal, MD
St. Albans, N.Y.

1996—Randall C. Morgan, Jr., MD, MBA
Gary, Ind.

1997—Nathaniel H. Murdock, MD, FACOG
St. Louis, Mo.

1998—Gary C. Dennis, MD, FAANS, FACS
Washington, D.C.

1999—Walter W. Shervington, MD
New Orleans, La.

2000—Javette C. Orgain, MD, MPH, FAAFP, Chicago, Ill.

2000—Rodney G. Hood, MD, FACP
San Diego, Calif.

2001—Lucille C. Norville Perez, MD
Bethesda, Md.

2002—L. Natalie Carroll, MD

Houston, Texas

2003—Randall W. Maxey, MD, PhD
Houston, Texas

2004—Winston Price, MD, FAAP, FACPE
Brooklyn, N.Y.

2005—Sandra L. Gadson, MD
Flossmoor, Ill.

2006—Albert W. Morris, Jr., MD
Memphis, Tenn.

2007—Nelson L. Adams, III, MD
Miami, Fla.

2008—Carolyn Barley Britton, MD, MS
New York, N.Y.

2009—Willarda V. Edwards, MD, MBA
Baltimore, Md.

2010—Leonard Weather, Jr., RPH, MD
Shreveport, La.

2011—Cedric M. Bright, MD, FACP
Durham, N.C.

2012—Rahn Kennedy Bailey, MD, FAPA
Nashville, Tenn.

2013—Michael LeNoir, MD
Oakland, Calif.

Rahn Kennedy Bailey, MD,
113th President, National Medical Association

Rahn K. Bailey, MD, DFAPA was installed as the 113th President of the National Medical Association (NMA) in July 2012. Dr. Bailey is chairman of the Department of Psychiatry at Meharry Medical College in Nashville, Tenn.

Dr. Bailey earned his doctorate degree from the University of Texas Medical Branch in Galveston in 1990. He completed his residency in psychiatry at the University of Texas at Houston and Texas Medical Center Affiliated Hospital, and he was chief resident from 1993 to 1994. He then served a fellowship in forensic psychiatry in the Department of Psychiatry at Yale University in New Haven, Conn. in 1995.

Dr. Bailey has held assistant professor clinical teaching positions at University of Texas Medical Center in Houston, Baylor College of Medicine in Houston, Louisiana State University Medical Center and Tulane in New Orleans, La. He was promoted to associate professor at University of Alabama at Birmingham Medical Center.

He is certified in general psychiatry (1998, re-certified 2008) and forensic psychiatry (1999, re-certified 2010) by the American Board of Psychiatry and Neurology. He has 31 peer-reviewed articles, 13 invited articles and two book chapter published.

Dr. Bailey is a member of several professional medical societies. He has received a variety of academic awards and honors, including the Chester M. Pierce, MD, ScD, Resident Research Award (1995) and the National Medical Association (NMA) Postgraduate

Physician Section Award (1998). He was named Outstanding Faculty by the University of Texas Medical School in Houston (2000), Region V Physician of the Year by the National Medical Association (2006) for his exemplary efforts in coordinating medical care for victims of Hurricane Katrina. Dr. Bailey was the most recent recipient of the Isaac Slaughter Memorial Leadership Award (2010).

In May, 2013, Dr. Bailey was unanimously elected to the Alpha Omega Alpha Honor Medical Society Gamma Chapter of Tennessee. Alpha Omega Alpha is a national professional medical organization that recognizes and advocates for excellence in scholarship and the highest ideals in the profession of medicine.

He served as President-Elect of the National Medical Association (2011-2012), Deputy Representative to the American Psychiatric Association from the Black Caucus of the APA, President-Elect of the Tennessee Psychiatric Association (May 2010-2011) and President (May2011-2012).